Defeat Your Skinny Genetics – Transform To Muscular

SAIANAND RAMAN

Introduction – Mission Transformation

Every 'body' has its own nature. And transformation of that body nature is a multi-dimensional process. That is one exercise regimen doesn't yield results to all. One diet regimen doesn't yield results to all. So the mystery is, what unique regimen will transform your body? This book will reveal the mystery thereby helping you to discover your own regimen to construct your body. What is required of you is the fighting spirit to travel against the wind, that is you need to fight to alter your skinny genetic programming. It could even be said you need a revolutionary mind set to create a revolution in your body. Good news is that, it is possible to redesign/reconstruct your body.

World Health Organization's definition of Health:

Health is a complete state of physical, mental and social well-being and not merely an absence of disease or infirmity.

Is it worth the efforts?

Right or wrong, almost everyone judges a book by its cover, though many preach otherwise. Similarly almost everyone judges/perceives/decides a person mainly (I used the word 'mainly' instead of 'absolutely', because some may not be willing to acknowledge and accept, what they practice is not what they preach) by his/her physical appearance.

Hence it will not be an overstatement to say that once 'Self-Esteem' is majorly impacted by his/her physical appearance. Because physical appearance is an omnipresent feature of the self, always on display for others or for the self to observe and evaluate. In contrast, one's adequacy in such domains as scholastic and athletic competence, peer likability, behavioral conduct, or morality is not constantly on display for evaluation. The world neither has the time nor patience to take pains in knowing who you really are? It's easy for them to go by, what is readily available on display.

Given the intangible but real importance given to physical appearance, nobody in this world can question a person's need based desire to improve his/her physical appearance in whatever way possible. And nobody can discount a person's efforts in this regard.

Hence if you want to pursue your need/desire to improve your physical appearance thereby your self-esteem, you are entitled to do so, and your efforts in this regard is by no means lesser to a person's need to pursue rocket science. In fact the efforts, dedication, determination, vigor, unrelenting attitude required to transform a skinny body to muscular is more challenging than understanding rocket science.

If pursuing your need based desire can help you achieve the following things mentioned below, never hesitate to pursue your need, go for it. You will never regret.

- Courage

- Peace of mind and Happiness

- Self-Esteem – Respect for you in your eyes

- Recognition & Respect – In the eyes of others (after all every human is a social animal, and requires some degree of approval, acceptance, importance from fellow human being, at-least from those few whom he/she considers important)

- Enthusiasm in life (Life is where enthusiasm is)

- Social Aliveness (Removal of inhibitions/barriers arising from social anxiety)

- Complete holistic life filled with experiences, adventures, joy of living, exploration, excitement, liveliness

Table of Contents

Gradually fight body's resistance to change

As we human resist any kind of change, our body too by nature highly resists change. Hence guide your body to gradually accept change. That is, let your muscles feel different workouts for various parts of the body like chest, shoulder, biceps, triceps, lats, and legs.

For first 4 to 6 months let your muscle get accustomed to different exercises. Get the help of trainer, internet exercise videos etc to perform the exercises with right technique. Learning to do the exercises without getting your muscles injured is of foremost importance. In this stage increasing the weight of dumbbell/barbell must be gradual because just increasing weights without doing the workouts with perfect technique limits the improvement.

Keep your motivation intact, even if you feel the signs of development in not visible enough. You need to accept the fact that transformation from skinny to muscular cannot be done in a few months' time. But always believe that the process towards the great transformation of your body has begun.

Gradually fight body's resistance to change

This is the stage of invisible improvements and foundation for visible development.

It will be useful to note that for persons with skinny body type it will be advantageous to do physical activity in the evening time, as you will have good energy level as a result of your healthy lunch. Morning time exercise is effective for stout people to burn fat.

Make use of all the available equipment's like dumbbell, barbell, cable, and freehand exercises. Don't neglect any exercise because you feel it's difficult, just trying persistently is what is required. For example, many find it difficult to do pull-ups and quit after 2 or 3 attempts. But a beginner should repeatedly try, just try pull-ups for at-least a month continuously in-order to see & feel the improvement.

Don't let muscles rest in comfort zone

This is a stage where you need to involve your body to variety of physical movements. The motive of this is to intentionally break the comfort zone of muscles. When you feel your body is getting used to workouts you do in the gym, involve your muscles in endurance training activities like swimming, aerobics, running, cycling etc one after the other. This is a way to get each and every muscles of the body to strengthen gradually without getting used to any one form of physical activity.

The importance of this stage is that, you ensure your muscles do not get accustomed to just one routine, that is breaking a routine and bringing in variety thereby getting your muscles experience different forms of physical activity will help muscles to evolve.

Exploring with variety of physical activity is a critical step in the process of body transformation. The motive behind this step is similar to sowing different variety of seeds in a land, in-order to keep the land healthy & vibrant.

Don't let muscles rest in comfort zone

Once the muscles of your body get vibrant, it means the body transformation process has gained momentum. You will feel energetic in this stage and you will begin to gradually understand the language of muscles. That is how your muscles interact and responds to different forms of physical activities.

This means, the stage is set for the great transformation from skinny to muscular.

Understand the chain reaction

It is better to understand early that your muscles are not a separate entity which is completely unrelated to the other functions of the body. On the contrary each and every functions of the body are deeply interrelated. That is transformation of body is a comprehensive process and should be looked in totality. In-order to transform your body physical activities play a vital role, but concentrating on physical activities alone excluding proper diet, rest, lifestyle, clean habits free of alcohol, smoking, and last but important having a healthy positive mind free of stress, anxiety are all important to the overall transformation process.

Focusing on one aspect by neglecting others will not yield the desired result. That is body transformation is a chain reaction, disturbing or neglecting one will automatically have impact on the others in that chain. Hence it is imperative to give equal importance to every aspect of the transformation process. Needless to say everything goes hand in hand, proper exercise needs proper diet which in-turn requires good

Understand the chain reaction

rest which needs proper lifestyle and habits which requires good mind frame.

In this stage you can put yourself in the self-examination mode to check which part of the chain is not in alignment with the desired mission. And take corrective measures as and when you find non-alignment in-order to ensure your mission flows smooth without unnecessary and avoidable hindrances.

Experiment to find your unique regimen

You will be entering this stage with some knowledge on techniques of doing exercises the right way and how your muscles respond to workouts. Now it's time to put those knowledge to optimum use in finding your unique workout regimen.

This is a stage for exploration because you have got your muscles perfectly tuned to accept different forms of physical activities and to reciprocate positively. Hence you need to get your muscles perform variety of workouts both weight training and endurance training.

In weight training you can use variety to train different parts of your body like chest, shoulders, biceps, triceps, legs, and lats. For example, if you take chest workouts, you can do it using dumbbell, barbell/rod and hydraulic machines/cable which provides variety to your workouts and also let your muscles explore different arena to development. In addition rotating your workouts helps in preventing lethargy which may set it after some time as a result of following the same routine always.

Experiment to find your unique regimen

Also use this stage to improvise your workouts to extract the best out of the workout. Even slight improvisation like changing the position of your grip could change the feel of the workouts but remember to always do workouts with right techniques. Improvisation should not compromise the technique. Once you have gained experience in doing workouts you will know by yourself how to improvise workouts to your advantage. It's a learning you will gain out of experience which could not be taught by trainers.

It is useful to know that workouts performed using dumbbell and barbell are helpful in improving your muscle size. Workouts using hydraulic machines/cable are helpful in getting your muscles in shape. Free hand exercises like pull-ups, push-ups, dips etc serves you best in increasing power. Free squat, Jumping squat, running will help you to increase stamina.

The motive of any experiment is to get the desired result. The motive of experimenting with different workouts is to find your unique regimen. Those workouts, that interacts perfectly with your muscles and responds with muscle improvement.

Performance Enhancers to break Genetic Shackles

The disadvantage with persons with skinny body type is that you find the muscle interactions with different physical activities though cordial doesn't translate to transformation. The reason behind this mystery is that, the genetic code of skinny person is a tough nut to crack.

In such a case you need not get disheartened being unable to break the shackles which inhibit your transformation. This is where performance enhancers serve as critical aid in breaking the unrelenting genetic structure. It's not a bad idea to get opinion from your family physician before starting with performance enhancers.

Some performance enhancers useful for your mission are Creatine monohydrate powder, Amino Acid tablets, Whey protein powder. Buy only from reputed manufacturers who are in business for a period of time. Don't buy from fly by night buyers. Exert caution in choosing and using performance enhancers.

Performance Enhancers to break Genetic Shackles

Creatine Monohydrate:

This is a performance enhancer which will kick open your genetic door. Exert caution in using creatine. Take creatine just for 3 months, with a serving of just 5 grams per day. It is better to take it by mixing with grape juice one hour before your workout. Creatine increases your energy level exponentially. It is your duty to put that huge energy increase to best use. And while using creatine drink plenty of water, say 5 liters per day. This is the stage where you need to hit the peak in weight training, as you will possess extreme energy to do heavy weight lifting. As you would have found your unique exercise regimen by the end of previous stage, it is imperative to attain peak in your unique regimen with the help of creatine.

Remember to use performance enhancers one after other. That is, use creatine for 3 months and then stop using. Give 2 months break before starting your next enhancer. Then take whey protein for 3 months and then stop.

Performance Enhancers to break Genetic Shackles

Give a break for 2 or 3 months before starting amino acids. Use amino acids for 2 or 3 months and put a permanent stop to using supplements/performance enhancers.

You should not live on performance enhancers. The motive of using performance enhancers is only to defeat your skinny genetic shackles and not beyond that. You need to know that performance enhancers are not natural organic substances and hence don't get carried away by its substantive energy effects. Always remember the motive of using it.

Always keep in mind, these performance enhancers are not replacement for healthy natural diet. It is highly recommended to use these enhancers intermittently for about a year and then stop it and continue with your regular natural healthy diet to maintain the gains achieved through performance enhancers.

Plough your body

This stage is about evolving from good to great and that is what transformation is. The general saying says, that which changes (positively), develops and that which changes often, transforms greatly. This is exactly what you should do with your muscles, at this stage.

You need to exploit your physical resources to its optimum best. Resources you have naturally and resources you gained through workouts and resources which the performance enhancers provided you, all of these resources must be exploited to the core.

Here you need to plough your body with all the resources you gained. What I mean by ploughing the body is, you need to make muscles experience unexplored training activities. As stated earlier your muscles should not be allowed to rest in comfort zone. If the muscles feel very much comfortable with a workout, it means it is time to alter workouts, change routines or even shift to different physical activity for a brief period after which you can return again to weight training. For example if you have been doing weight training for over a year, give a small break for say 3 or 4 months and get your muscles to experience swimming activity. If you feel you have more energy which is available for an additional activity, you can even combine weight training with swimming simultaneously. Similarly you can shift or combine other endurance activities like aerobics, yoga, running for a brief period of time, which will serve as rejuvenation. Whenever you get a sense that your muscle feels the workouts monotonous or enjoying more comfort in an activity, it's time for a brief shift before you get back to weight training.

The principle behind this approach is similar to that of sowing seeds in a land. That is, just one type of seed will not be sowed continuously in a land, instead different varieties of seeds are sown. This type of rotating the seeds in cycle helps the land to remain highly fertile always. The same principle is applied by sowing the body with variety of activities so that muscles remain vibrant for transformation.

By now your body would have transformed to what you were dying for. Mission transformation is achieved in this stage.

Diet – Find what works

First and foremost it important to demolish the commonly believed myth that the one and only reason why skinny people remain how they are, is because they don't eat the right quality and quantity of healthy food. The fact is, they are how they are, is majorly due to genetic factors. Specifically the genetic disadvantage of fast metabolism can be fixed with the help of performance enhancers.

As stated in the earlier part of this book that, 'One exercise regimen doesn't fit all' similarly one diet which works for your friend or others need not work the same way to produce the same results as that of your friend, as your body nature is totally different from his or her. So you need to find what diet works for you to bring about transformation of your body.

You need to increase intake of healthy calories, that's a must. But how to do that in a comfortable way instead of force feeding yourself against your body's command needs to be explored. Let's begin with some basic information on nutrition & diet. Protein which is known as the muscle builder is a vital component in achieving your mission.

Diet – Find what works

The body breaks protein into amino acids for absorption. But narrowing your focus on protein alone neglecting carbohydrates and fats will not help you much. It is important to know carbohydrates and fats are necessary to replenish your energy system. Hence your diet should be proportionately balanced giving equal importance to protein, carbohydrates, fats and other vitamins.

Also in the process of finding your right diet, you need not give up your routine healthy foods which you have been following from childhood/which is an integral part of you. Instead you continue with your regular healthy diet but in addition fill up the nutritional gaps in your routine diet with enough protein, carbohydrates and fats.

The best way of increasing your calorie intake is to increase the number of times you eat in a day. That is, eat as and when you feel hungry, but ensure that you eat nutritious food instead of junk foods. You need not even give up your snacking habit. Just replace your stomach filling snacks without any nutritious value with snacks with nutritional value like protein bars, nuts, dry-fruits, milk/fruit shakes, cereal bars, soups or any other snacks which can satisfy both taste as well as nutritional requirements are fine. Finding your right diet regimen is not that difficult a process.

It is in your advantage to know that non-vegetarian foods are rich in quality protein compared to vegetarian foods. The quality protein consists of majority of amino acids. Hence it will be better for vegetarians to incorporate at-least certain non-vegetarian foods like egg, chicken, and fish if possible. Even if you could not incorporate the other non-vegetarian foods the above mentioned foods will greatly satisfy your protein requirements.

Remember to gradually increase your food intake, which will not be difficult as performing physical activities by itself will take care of increasing your appetite thereby increasing your intake.

Body-Mind connection

"The physiology of your body, determines the psychology of the mind".

I believe the world health organization's definition of health is the comprehensive definition of health. As per WHO, 'Health is a complete state of mental, social and physical well-being and not merely an absence of disease or infirmity.'

Few may be thinking, what is the role of mind in transformation of body. But the fact is body and mind are not two separate entities. Rather they are deeply interrelated/intertwined. To make it simple to understand, when someone is in anxiety his/her heartbeat increases, blood flow gets fast, adrenaline rush happens. When a person is in worry, there will be decrease/increase in appetite, decrease in quality sleep, weight loss/gain. All these changes are a result of hormonal reactions to the body initiated by the mind.

Some information about certain vital brain chemicals will be helpful to maintain positive frame of mind. Serotonin is a brain chemical also known as the feel-good chemical. Physical activities increase the production of serotonin by the brain. Oxytocin which is another brain chemical also called socializing chemical. And there is dopamine, a brain chemical which is also called the risk taking chemical. Endorphin is a brain chemical which helps in keeping pain and stress at bay. Proper production and balance of all these vital chemicals of the brain is of utmost importance in determining the quality of your life. Decrease in optimum levels of these critical brain chemicals will lead to depression, anxiety and other psychological problems.

When you are at the receiving end of the spectrum with regard to criticism, ridicule and other adversities of life, it will be difficult to maintain a positive mind frame. But you need to remember the importance of being positive even under difficult circumstances, because as stated earlier in this chapter, mind causes great impact on body. Your great mission of body transformation needs the support of mind without which the progress will be hindered. Only a positive mind will be free of/ will not be prone to fear, anxiety, worry, frustration, depression.

Hence I would suggest getting help from certain self-help and motivational books for maintaining positive mind frame by unweeding the train of negative thoughts. In this regard, I would personally suggest some titles which are,

If life is a game, these are the rules – author Cherie Carter-Scott (always get Indian edition of foreign author books which will cost less)

Whose life are you living – author Tony Humphreys

The monk who sold his Ferrari – Robin Sharma

The Alchemist – Paulo Coelho

Freedom from the known – J.Krishnamurti

Manase Relax please – Sukhabodhananda

Courage – The joy of living dangerously – Osho

If you are suffering from low self-esteem because of your physical characteristics/traits, I will strongly recommend the book titled,

Self-Esteem – Author Matthew McKay and Patrick Fanning, publisher Mastermind books, Vasan publications (Indian edition is low priced) – This book will bring earth shacking impact on you.

Yoga for Internal Transformation

The aid of yoga with regard to transforming body can be attributed mainly to four important functions, in addition to lots of other health and medical benefits.

First and foremost practicing yoga strengthens your breathing/respiratory system. The quality of your life is determined by the quality of your breath. By strengthening the respiratory system, yoga helps in free flow of oxygen throughout the body. An unhindered flow of oxygen is important for optimal absorption of nutrients by the body.

Yoga helps the lungs get full oxygen supply. More oxygen means improved health and energy. On the contrary shallow breathing leads to insufficient oxygen supply to the lungs which causes fatigue and an insufficient supply of oxygen due to weak respiratory system leads to lots of diseases. The body with more oxygen produces more energy.

The next important aid of yoga comes in the form of flexibility. Keeping your muscles flexible is important for the success of your mission. The room for growth of a rigid body is less compared to a flexible body. Hence it is important to keep your body flexible and yoga not only helps in maintaining the flexibility of your body but also strengthens your bones and keeps it healthy.

The next help from yoga comes in the form of rejuvenating/stimulating digestive system of your body. Practicing yoga increases your appetite through digestive system stimulation. This will automatically lead to good increase in food intake, which is a very important aspect of body transformation.

Yoga helps in balancing your hormone system, keeping it healthy, in perfect alignment with rest of the other body functions. For example an imbalance in thyroid hormone will inhibit growth similarly improper digestive system leads to improper absorption of nutrients you eat. Yoga helps to keeps your internal system of your body healthy and vibrant.

It is useful to understand that by keeping your breathing, digestive, hormone systems healthy and by increasing your appetite, quality of sleep and relaxing your muscles, yoga accelerates the momentum of success in your mission transformation.

The Physical Benefits of Yoga:

Performing yoga postures regularly offers a number of physical benefits, including:

- Increased flexibility

- Increased lubrication of joints, ligaments and tendons

- Massaging the body's internal organs

- Detoxifying the body

- Toning the muscles

Yoga postures and exercises focus on all of the joints of the body, including joints you probably don't use regularly. Yoga exercises can strengthen problem joints such as the knees, hips and ankles. Yoga training also leads to increased spinal flexibility and core strength, both of which can reduce chronic problems such as lower back pain and increase your overall physical strength. Because yoga also exercises ligaments and tendons, your joints will lubricate more effectively, reducing joint pain.

Yoga Anatomy – Effects on Muscles

Yoga training may be the only form of exercise that stimulates your internal organs. This helps prevent disease by maintaining organ health. It can also help make you more aware of potential health problems.

Yoga stretches and stimulates the muscles and organs of the body in a uniform manner. This allows increased blood flow to all parts of your body, which helps to flush out the toxins that can accumulate in your body's tissues. Increased detoxification can increase your energy levels

Note: It is better and advisable to learn the techniques of performing yoga, initially from a certified yoga trainer. Yoga course will be for around 3 months. After you learn the techniques, you can practice it at home/gym/ anywhere. After completing the 3 month yoga course, all you need is just a yoga mat and small space to perform it.

Yoga Anatomy with Pictures:

Jaanuseerasanam:

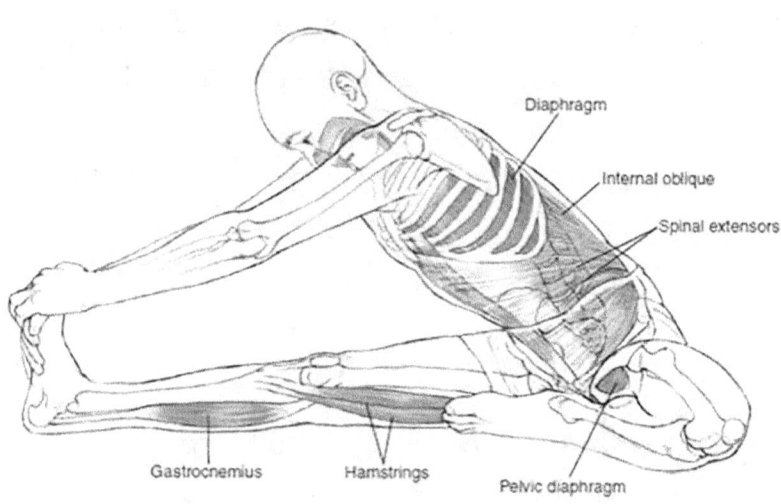

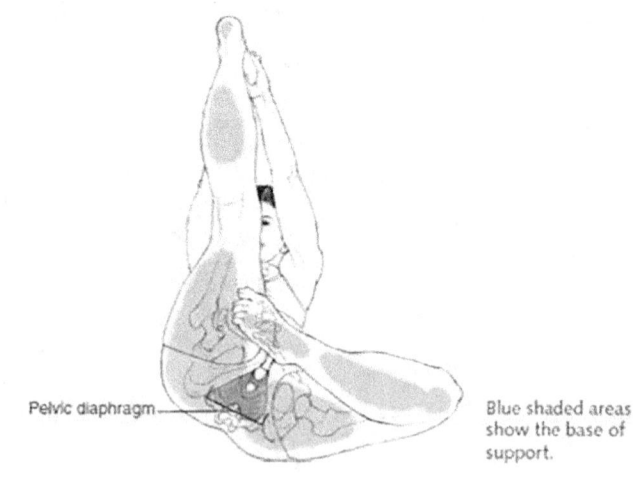

Paschimootasanam:

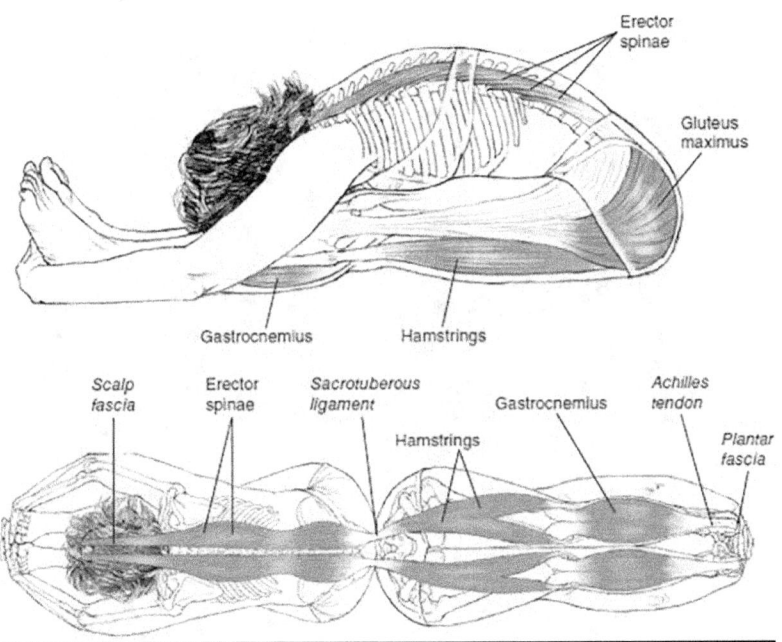

Navasanam:

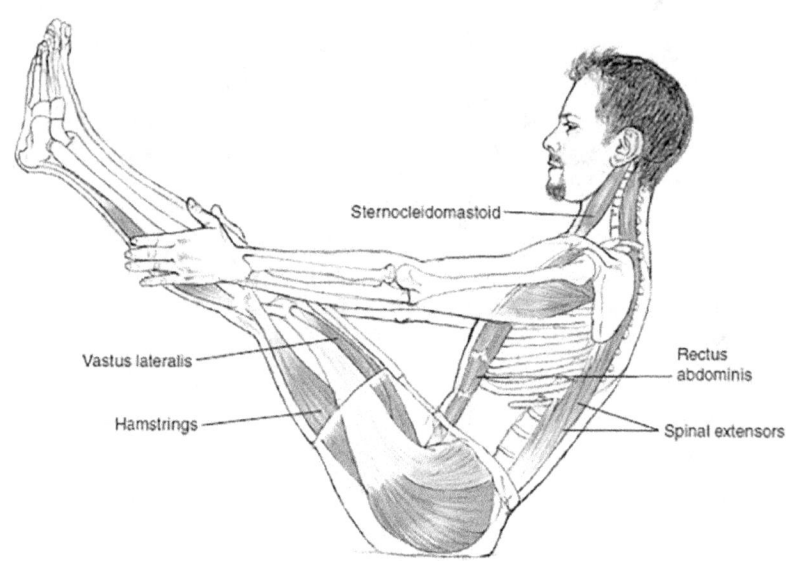

Supta-Vajrasanam:

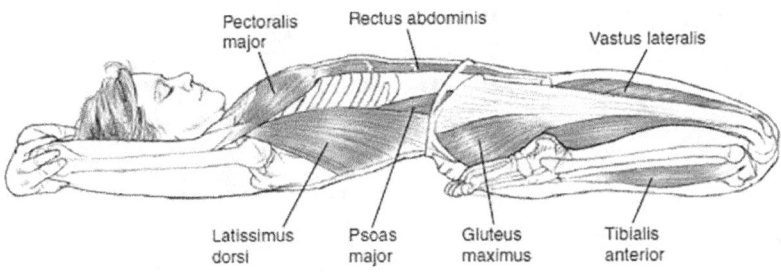

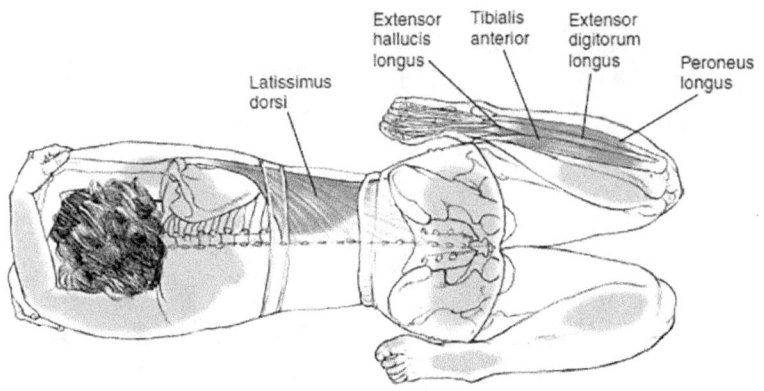

Bujangasanam:

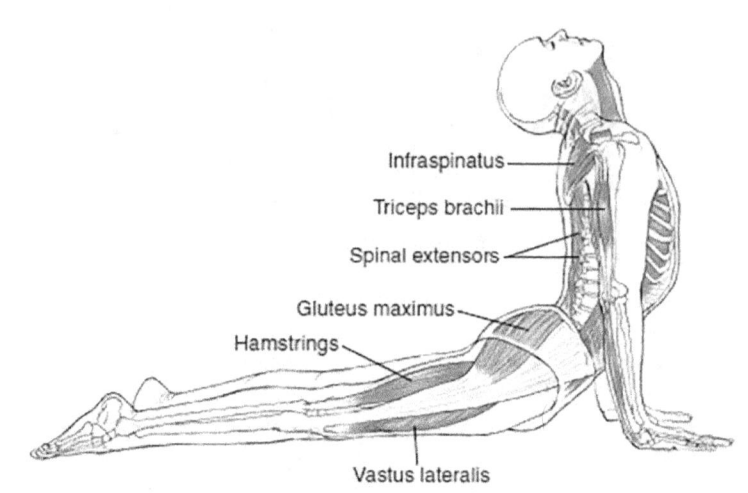

Infraspinatus

Triceps brachii

Spinal extensors

Gluteus maximus

Hamstrings

Vastus lateralis

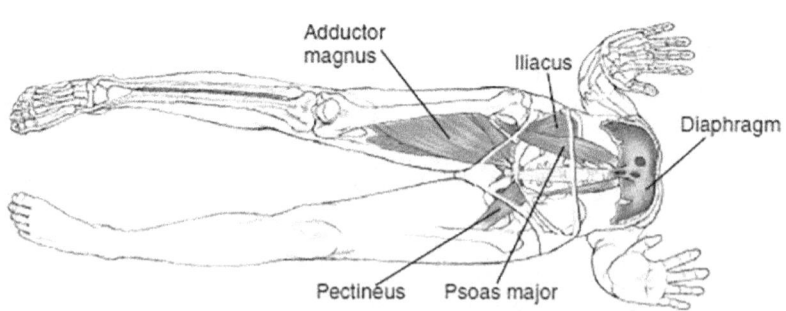

Adductor magnus

Iliacus

Diaphragm

Pectineus   Psoas major

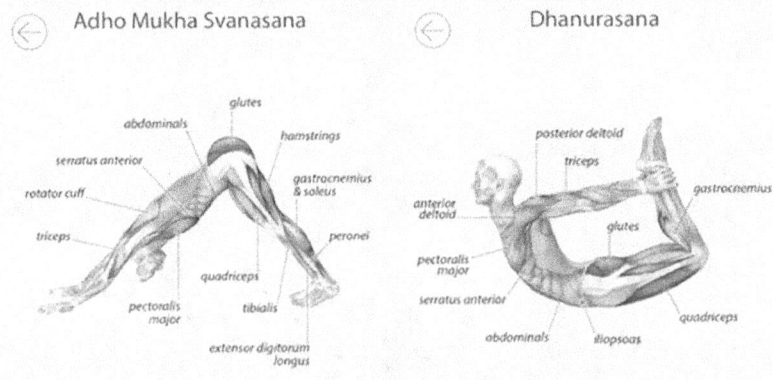

Adho Mukha Svanasana

glutes
abdominals
hamstrings
serratus anterior
gastrocnemius & soleus
rotator cuff
triceps
peronei
quadriceps
pectoralis major
tibialis
extensor digitorum longus

Dhanurasana

posterior deltoid
triceps
anterior deltoid
gastrocnemius
pectoralis major
glutes
serratus anterior
abdominals
iliopsoas
quadriceps

Dhanurasanam:

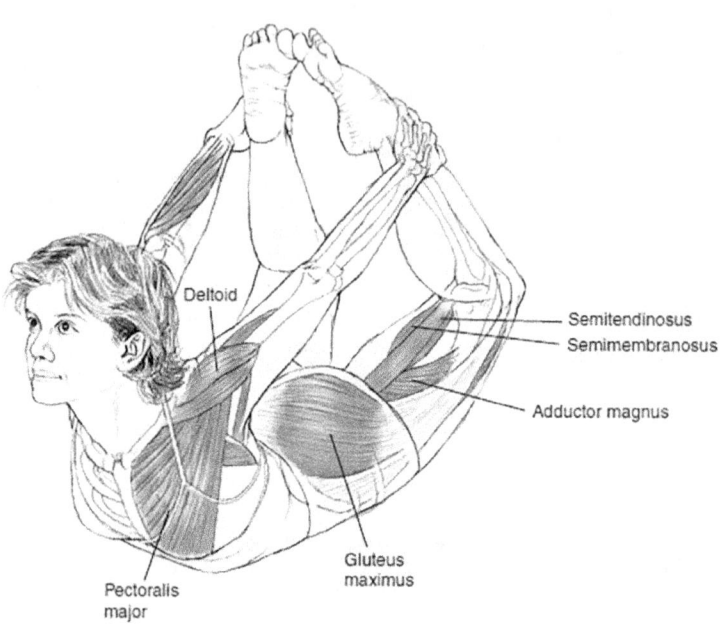

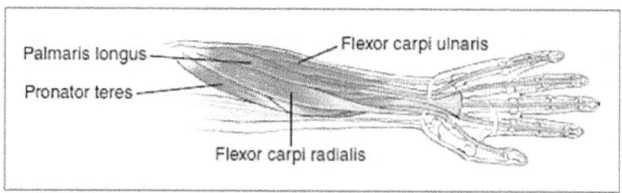

Halasanam:

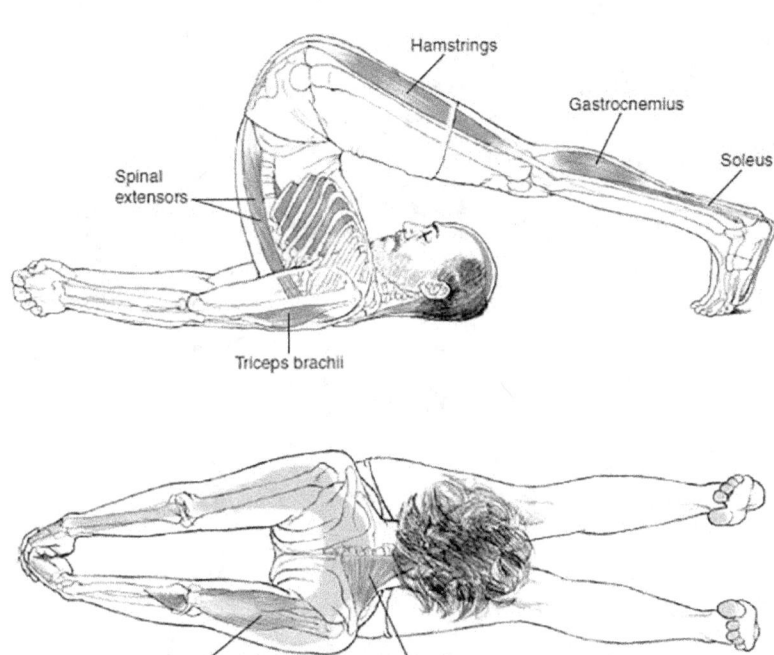

Sethubhandasanam – Position A:

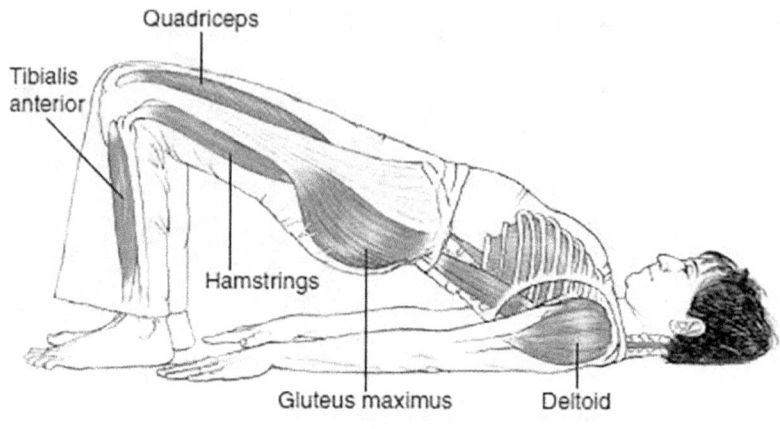

Inhalation.

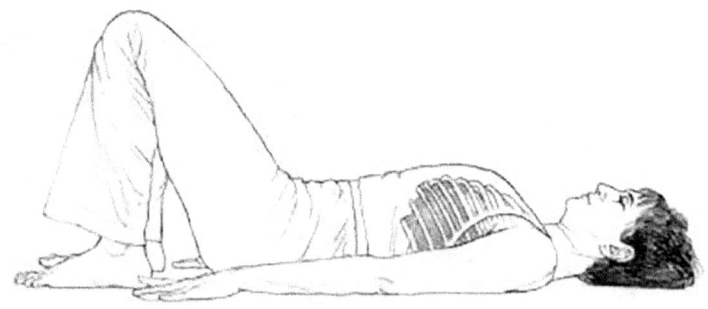

Exhalation.

Sethubhandasanam – Position B:

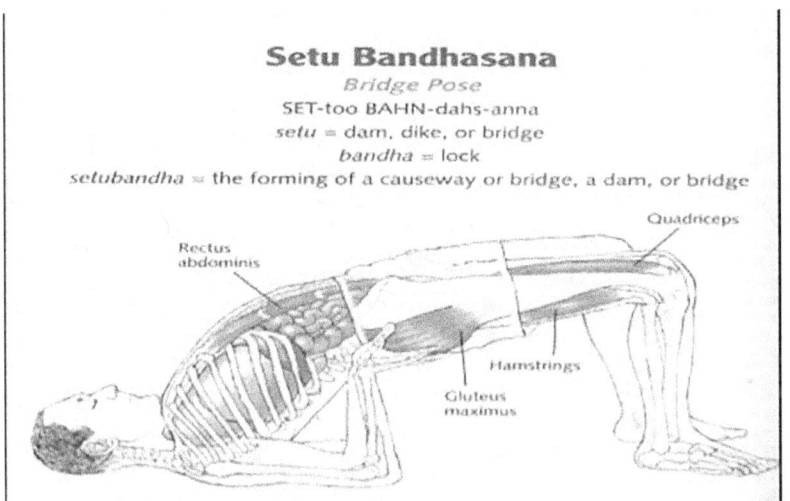

Setu Bandhasana

Bridge Pose

SET-too BAHN-dahs-anna

setu = dam, dike, or bridge

bandha = lock

setubandha = the forming of a causeway or bridge, a dam, or bridge

Quadriceps

Rectus
abdominis

Hamstrings

Gluteus
maximus

Purvottanasana:

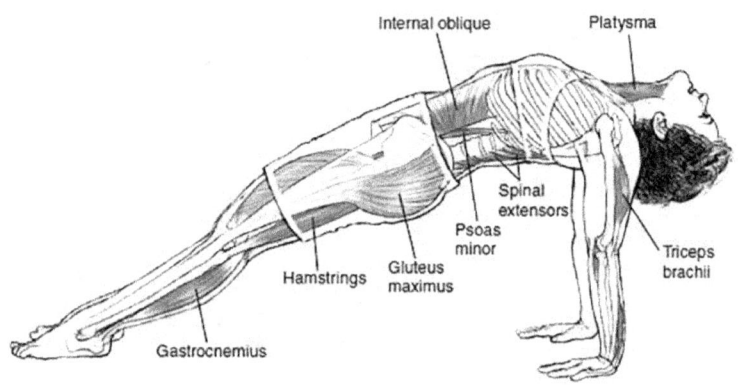

Usartaasana – Position A:

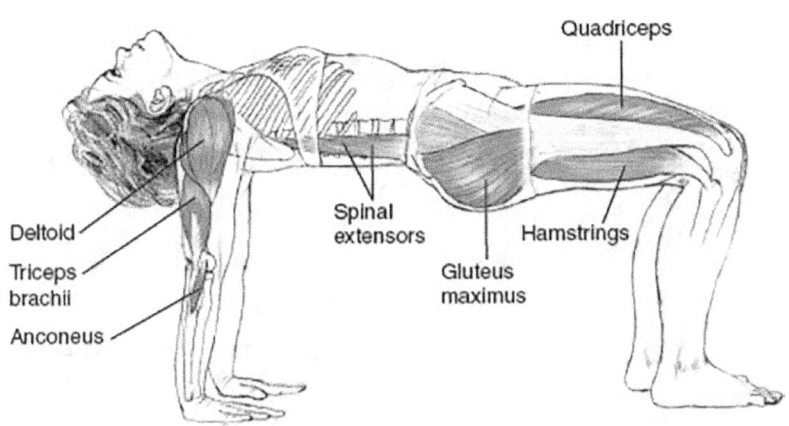

Quadriceps

Deltoid

Triceps brachii

Anconeus

Spinal extensors

Hamstrings

Gluteus maximus

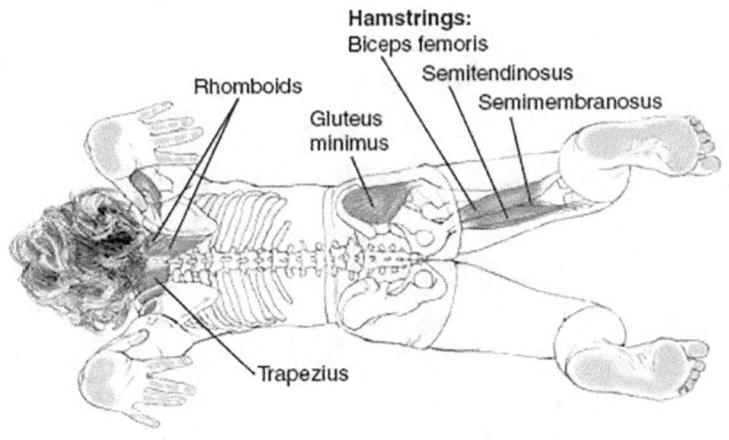

Hamstrings:
Biceps femoris
Semitendinosus
Semimembranosus

Rhomboids

Gluteus minimus

Trapezius

Usartaasana – Position B:

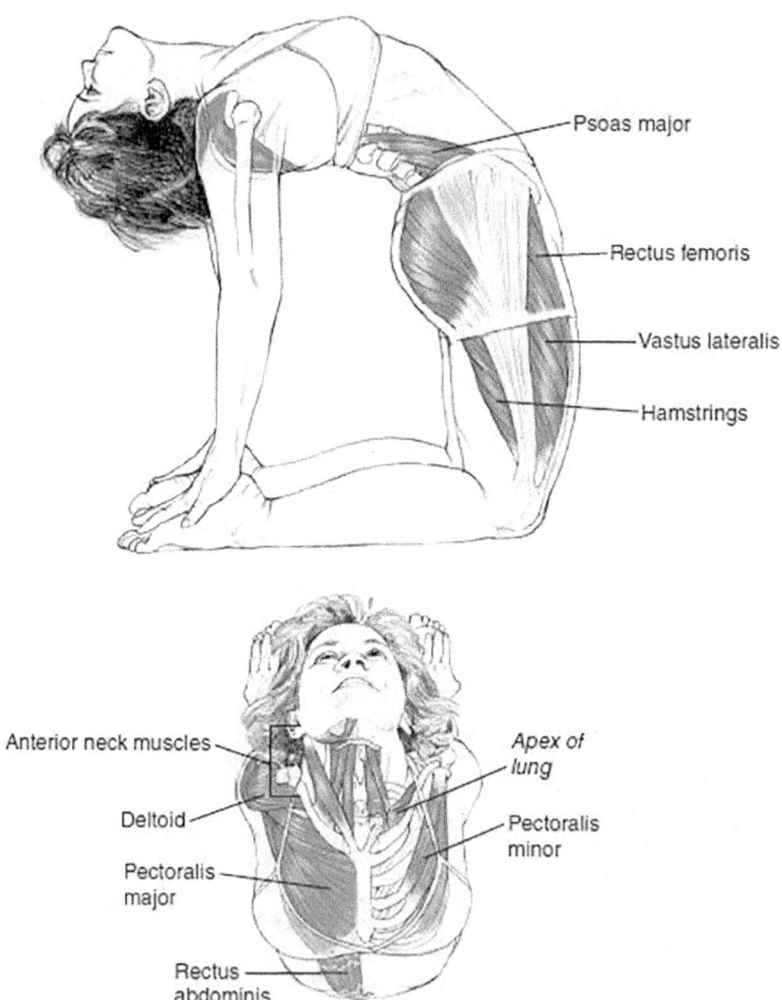

Psoas major

Rectus femoris

Vastus lateralis

Hamstrings

Anterior neck muscles

Apex of lung

Deltoid

Pectoralis minor

Pectoralis major

Rectus abdominis

Mayurasana:

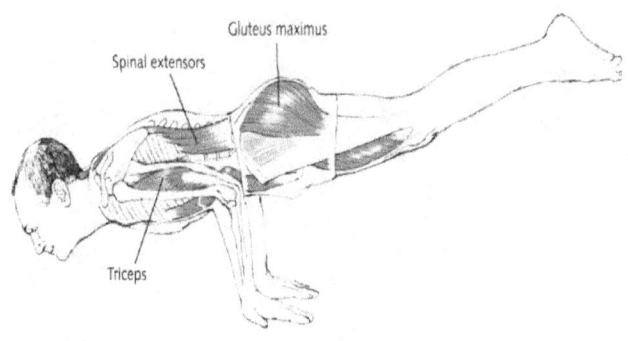

Chakrasana:

Wheel
Urdhva Dhanurasana

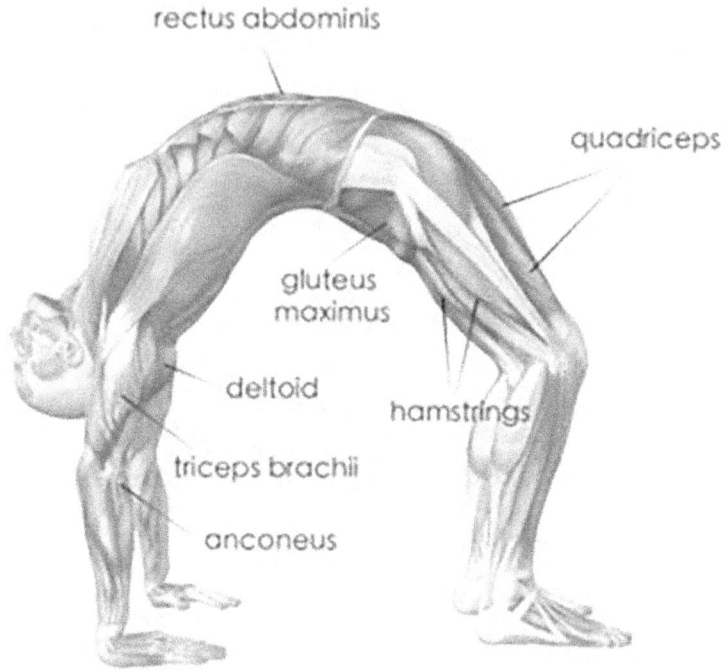

rectus abdominis

quadriceps

gluteus
maximus

deltoid

hamstrings

triceps brachii

anconeus

Contracting   Stretching

Sirasasanam:

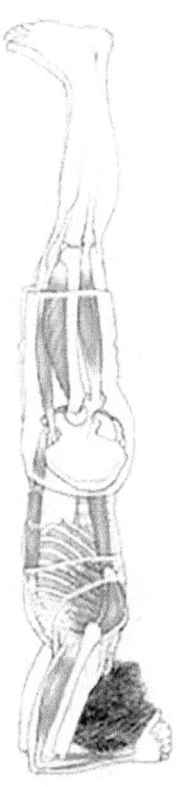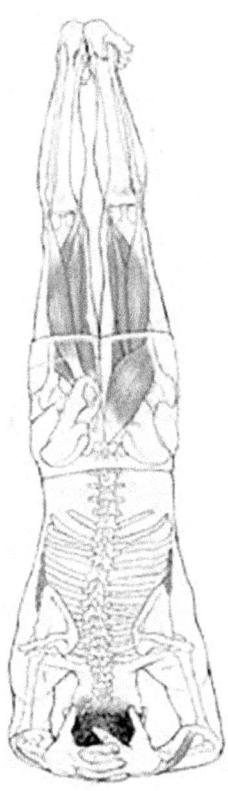

Shoulder Workouts:

Dumbbell Lying Rear Lateral Raise in Flat (or) Inclined bench:

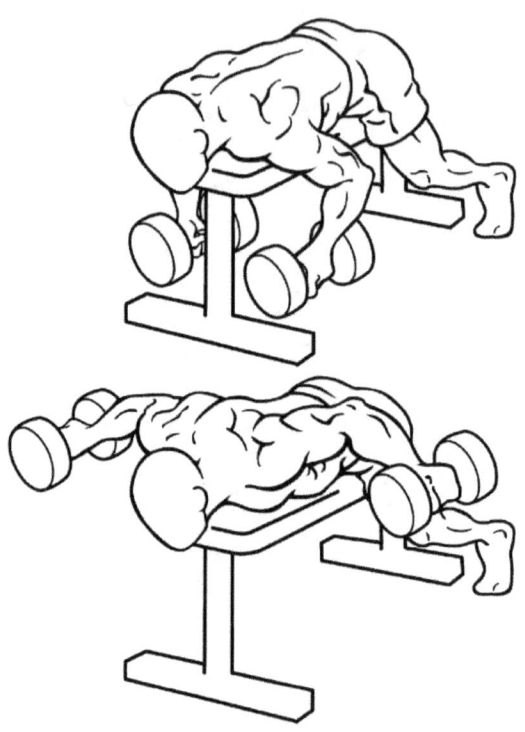

- While holding a dumbbell in each hand, lay with your chest/Face down on a flat bench. Make sure the bench is high enough so that the dumbbell does not touch the ground.

- Position the palms of the hands in a neutral manner (palms facing each other) as you keep the arms extended with the elbows slightly bent. This will be your starting position.

- Now raise the arms to the side until your elbows are at shoulder height and your arms are roughly parallel to the floor. Maintain your arms perpendicular to the torso while keeping them extended throughout the movement. Also, keep the contraction at the top for a second.

- Slowly lower the dumbbells to the starting position.

Variations: *Also you can perform this exercise with one arm, in flat bench and holding the frontal base of the bench with the other hand for balance.*

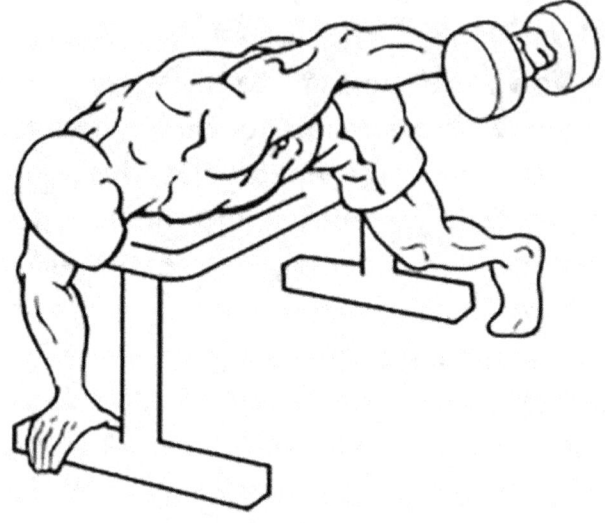

Lying Sideways Rear Deltoid Raise:

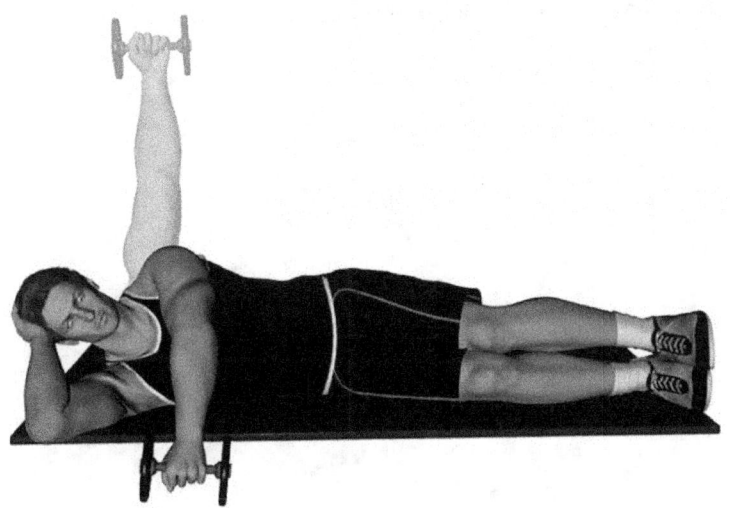

- Lay down on your side pressed in a flat bench, back and legs extended and hold a dumbbell with one hand, arms extended forward.

Uncommon but Effective Workouts

- Keep your non-training arm to clamp around the underneath of the bench with your upper leg leaning forward slightly off the edge.

- Raise the dumbbell out and up and slowly lower it back after a short pause.

Rear Deltoid Cable Fly:

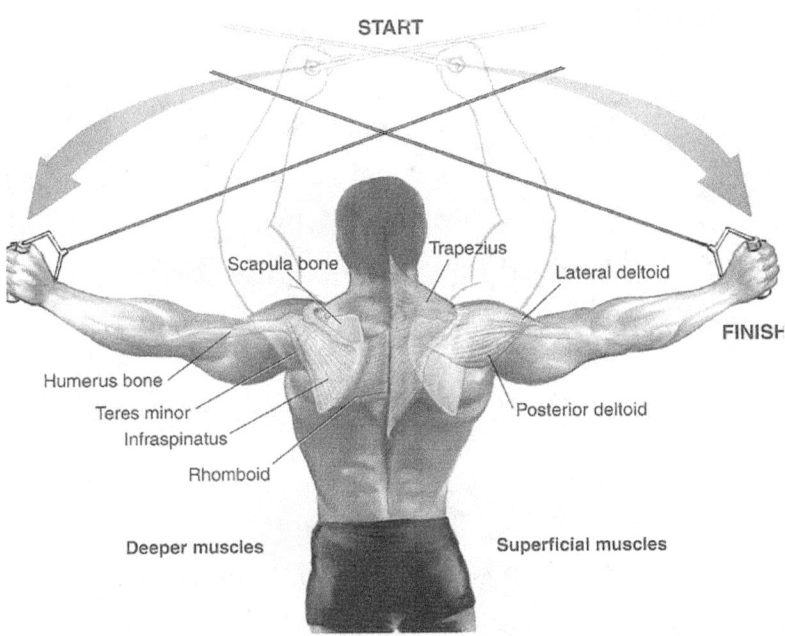

- Adjust the pulleys to the appropriate height and adjust the weight. The pulleys should be above your head.
- Grab the left pulley with your right hand and the right pulley with your left hand, crossing them in front of you. This will be your starting position.
- Initiate the movement by moving your arms back and outward, keeping your arms straight as you execute the movement.
- Pause at the end of the motion before returning the handles to the start position.

One Arm Incline Lateral Raise:

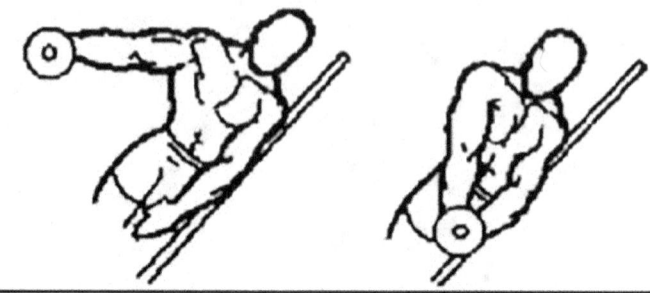

- Lay down on your side on a slightly inclined bench, set up at 45 degrees with a dumbbell in one hand. Make sure the shoulder is pressing against the incline bench and the arm is lying across your body.

- Raise the dumbbell up to where it is perpendicular to your torso – performing a lateral raise. Keep arm parallel to the floor.

- Squeeze at the top, so as to feel the contraction in the shoulder for 2 seconds.

- Lower the dumbbell across your body back into the starting position.

Front Incline Barbell/Dumbbell Raise:

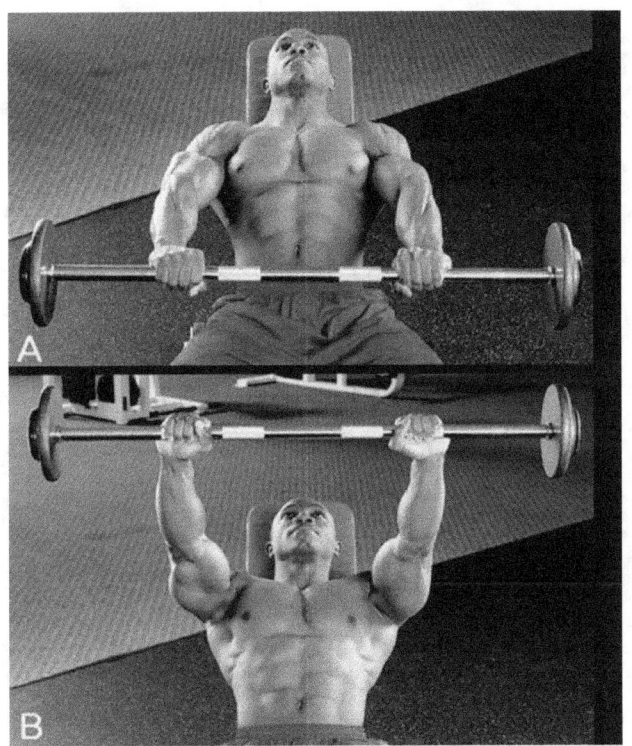

- Sit down on an incline bench with the incline set anywhere between 30 to 60 degrees while holding a light barbell with a shoulder width.

Note: *You can change the angle to hit the muscle a little differently each time.*

- Extend your arms straight in front of you and have your palms facing down with the barbell raised about 1 inch above your thighs. This will be your starting position.

- Slowly raise the barbell straight up until they are slightly above your shoulders, while keeping your elbows locked. Squeeze at the top for a second and make sure you breathe out during this portion of the movement. **Note:** Keep your head resting down against the bench and your legs on the floor at all times.

- Lower the arms back to the starting position.

Variations: *You can use Dumbbells as well for this exercise.*

Latissimus dorsi/Lats/Wings Workouts:

Pull-ups:

I personally believe, if there is one exercise that can be called, The King of all exercises, I can say without a second thought it would be the Pull-ups. The reason for saying so is, almost all the upper body muscles like lats, shoulder, biceps, triceps, forearms, abdomen are trained while doing pull-ups with different grips such as wide grip pull-ups, close grip pull-ups, reverse grip chin-ups, interlocking hands pull-ups, head/neck in front of bar pull-ups.

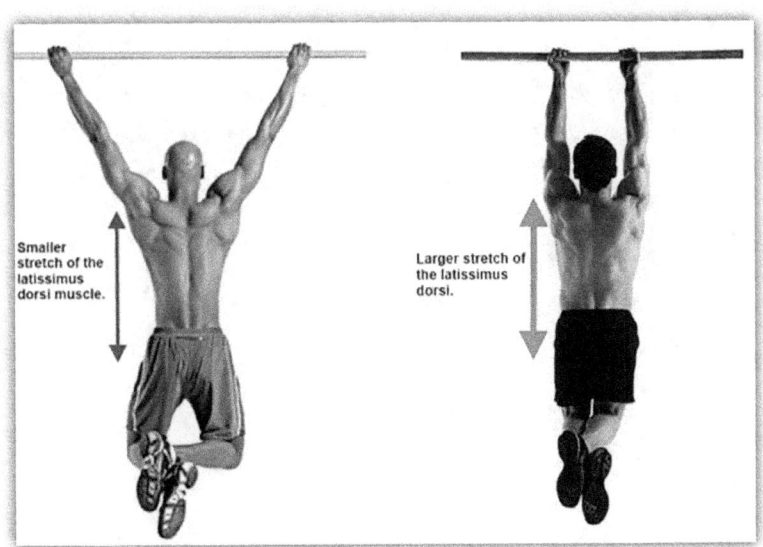

Smaller stretch of the latissimus dorsi muscle.

Larger stretch of the latissimus dorsi.

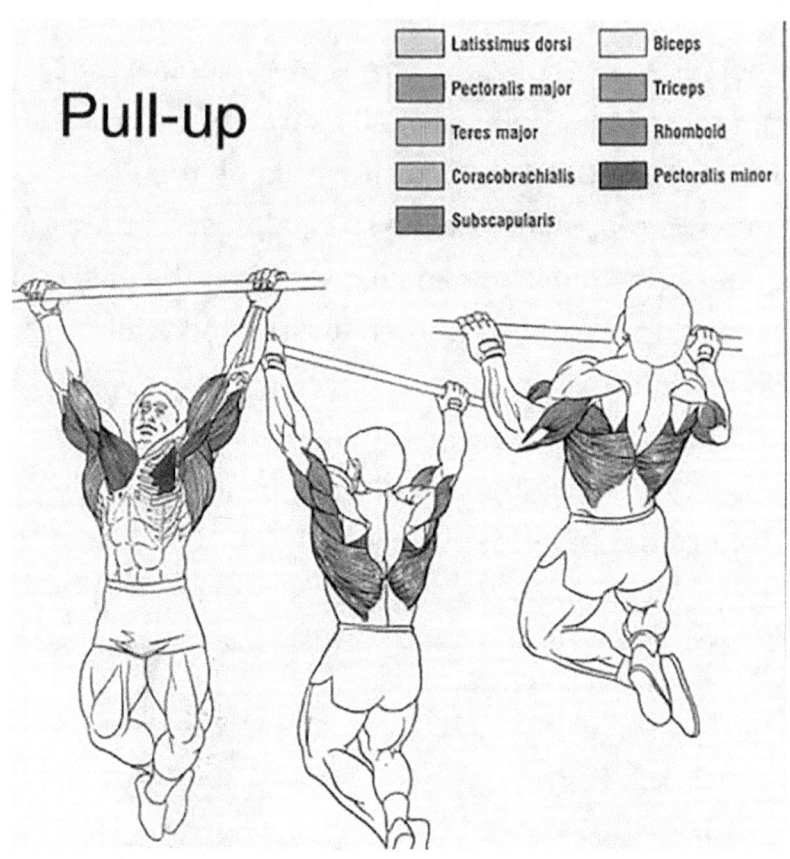

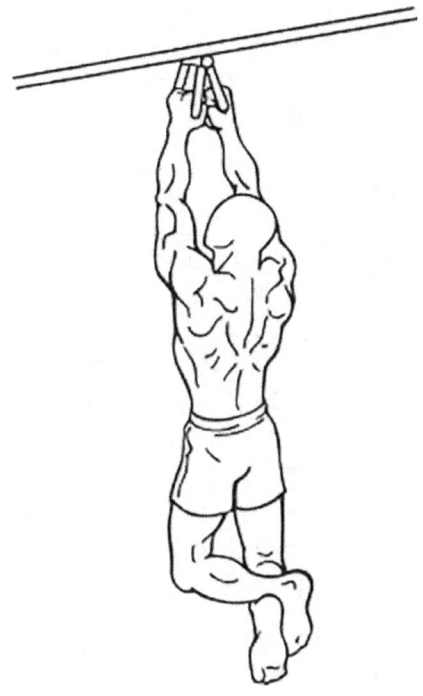

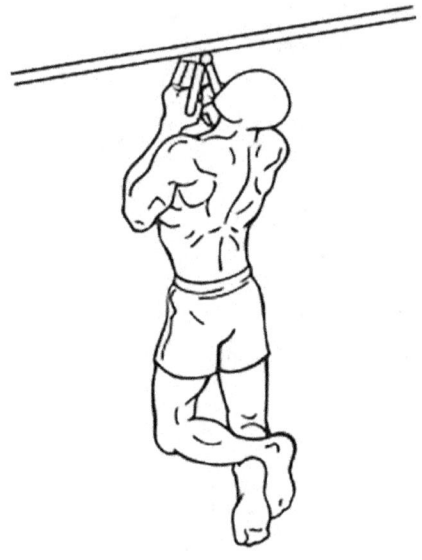

<u>Neck in front of the bar pull-ups</u>

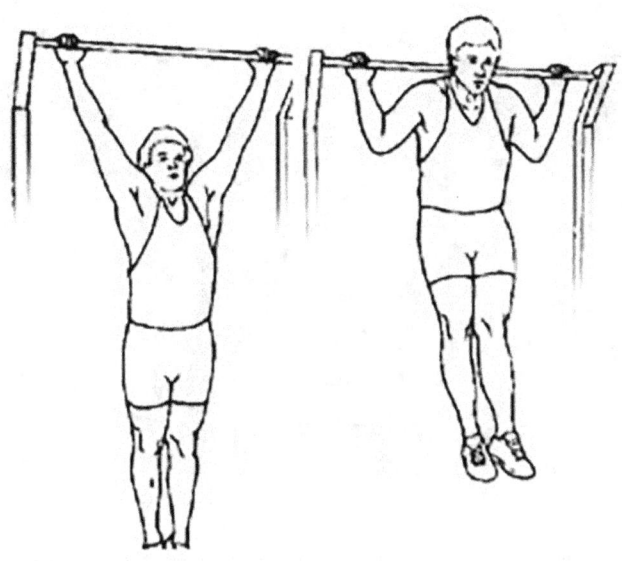

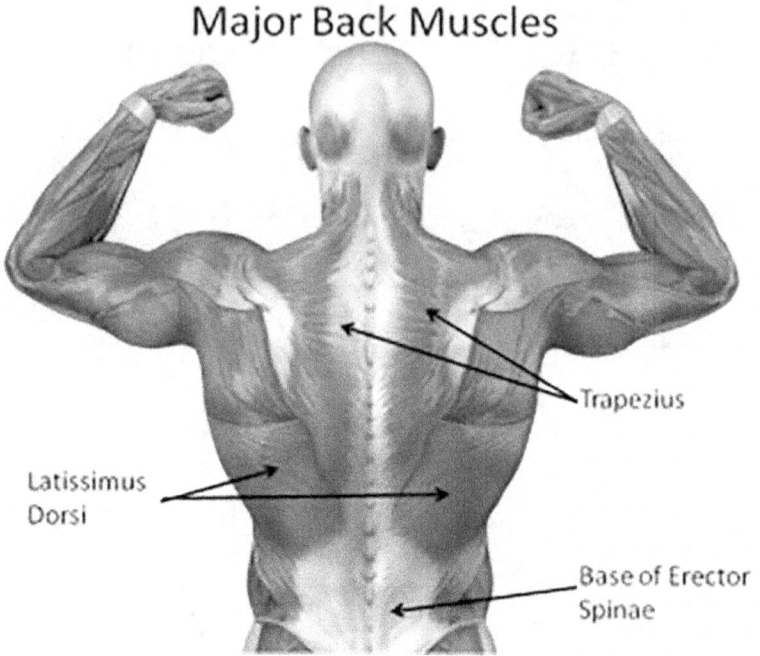

Major Back Muscles

<u>Pull-ups with weights:</u>

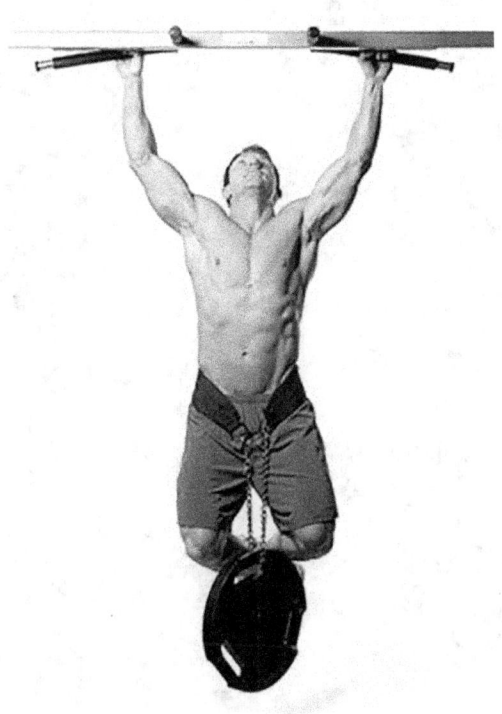

Kneeling down high pulley row with rope:

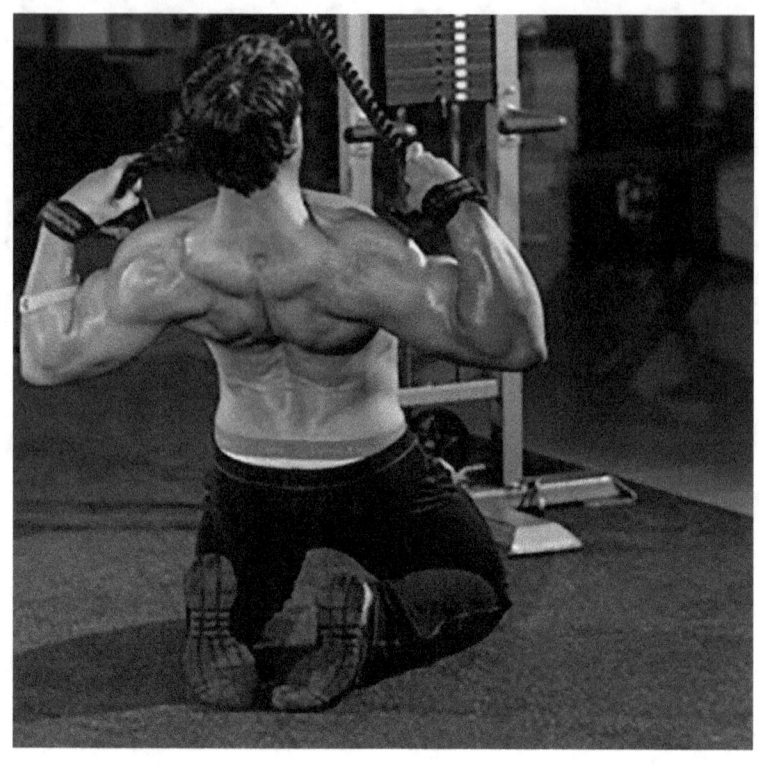

- Using a pulley that is above your head, attach a   rope to the cable and kneel a few feet away.

- Hold the rope out in front of you with both arms extended. This is your starting position.

- Flex your elbows and pull the rope toward your upper chest with your elbows out.

- After pausing briefly, slowly extend your elbows until your arms are fully extended.

Variation to Kneeling down high pulley row:

- *Kneel down and sit on your legs/calf, a few feet away from the pulley and bent forward making your abdomen closer to your thighs.*

- *Hold the rope and fully extend both your arms. This is your starting position.*

- *Pull the rope toward your upper chest and gradually stretch your arms back to the starting position similar to that of rowing boat action.*

Seated One-arm Cable Pulley Rows

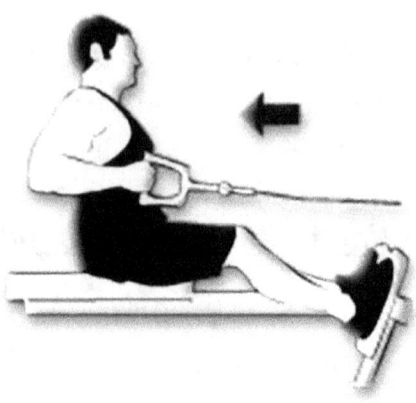

- Sitting on a seated row machine, reach forward and grab onto the handle attachment with one hand only.

- Sit up straight bending forward slightly at your hip with your back straight and head looking forward.

- Let the weight of the pulley bar attachment pull your arm straight with your palm facing in toward your body. This is the starting position.

- Pull the pulley bar attachment toward your upper abdomen until the attachment nearly touches your abdomen. This is the ending position.

- Return to the starting position by reversing the movement just performed.

- Repeat the same movement except this time with the other arm. Always perform the movement under control.

Variations:

You can perform this movement with a high pulley as well and standing up. Also you can perform this exercise in a half-kneeling position and you can perform it doing a full rotation of the wrist. In other words, at the starting position you will have the palms of the hands facing down and at the end of the movement they will be facing up.

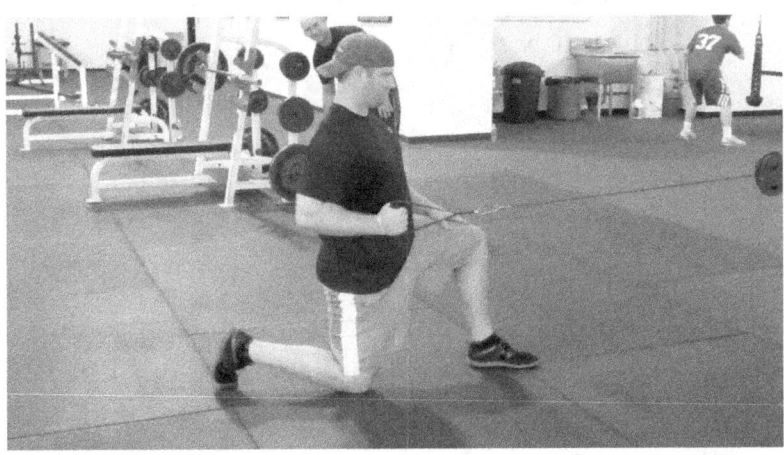

Dumbbell bend arm pullover:

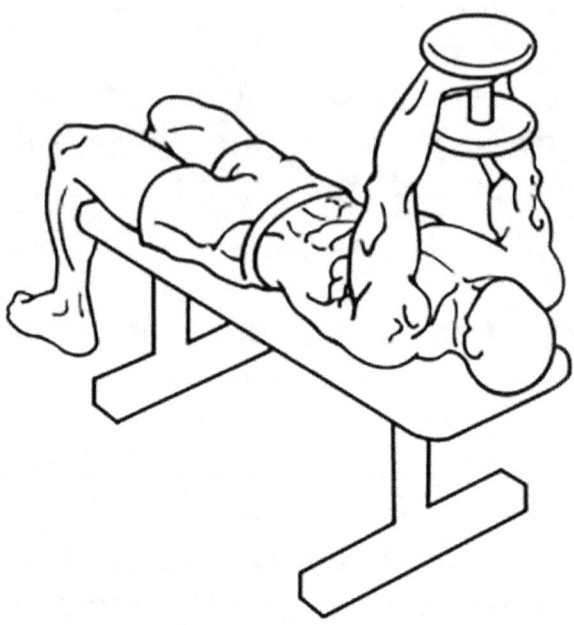

- Lie on a flat bench with your feet flat on the floor and your head at the end of the bench.

- Grasp a dumbbell and raise it over your chest.

- Keeping your elbows as straight as possible, lower the weight in an arc over your head and as low to the ground as possible without any pain.

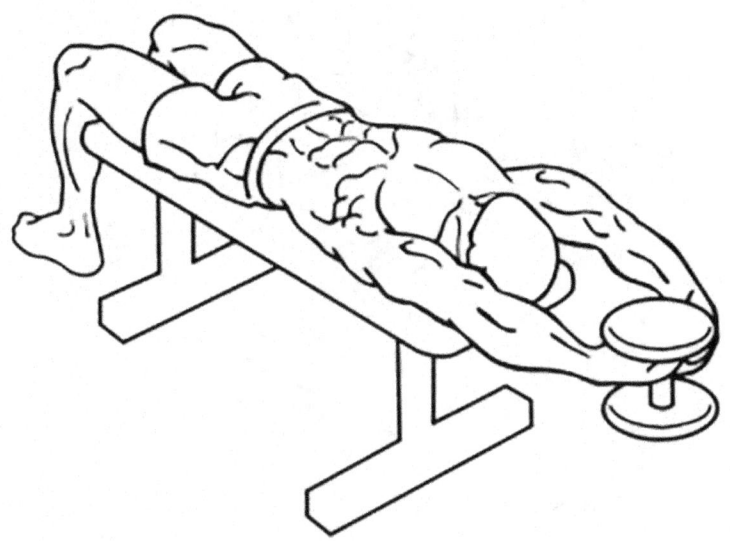

- Return to starting position.

Variations to this workout:

You can perform this workout with a barbell also. And you can also do it using an inclined bench.

Barbell bend arm pullover:

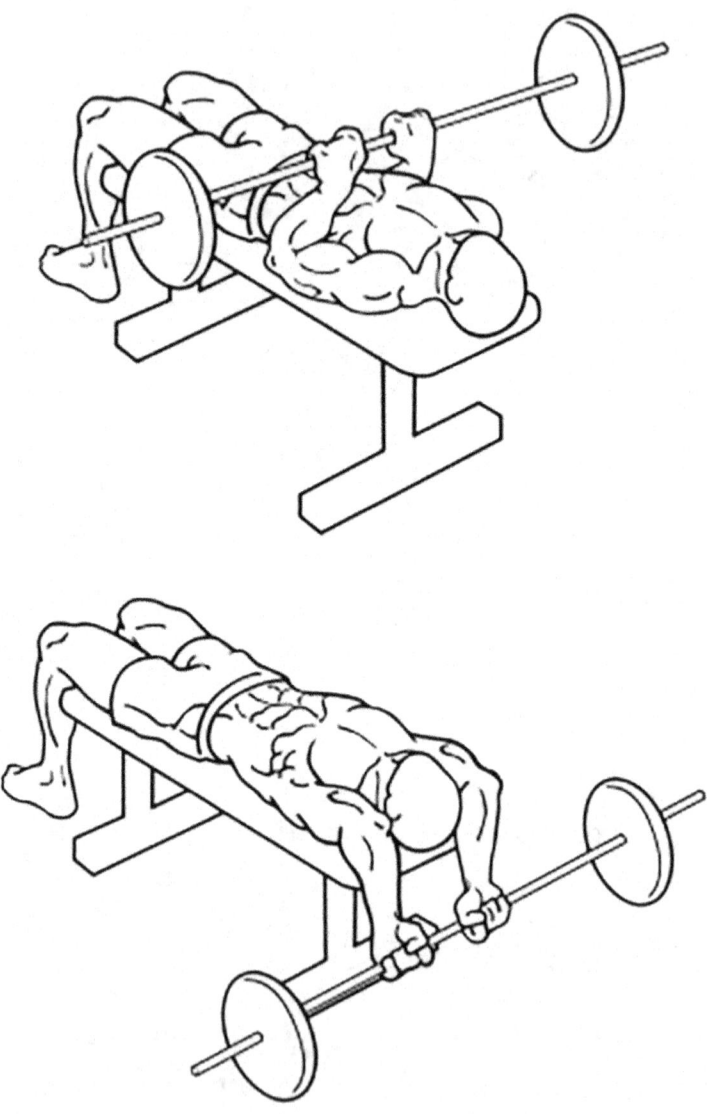

Bent over two arms long bar row:

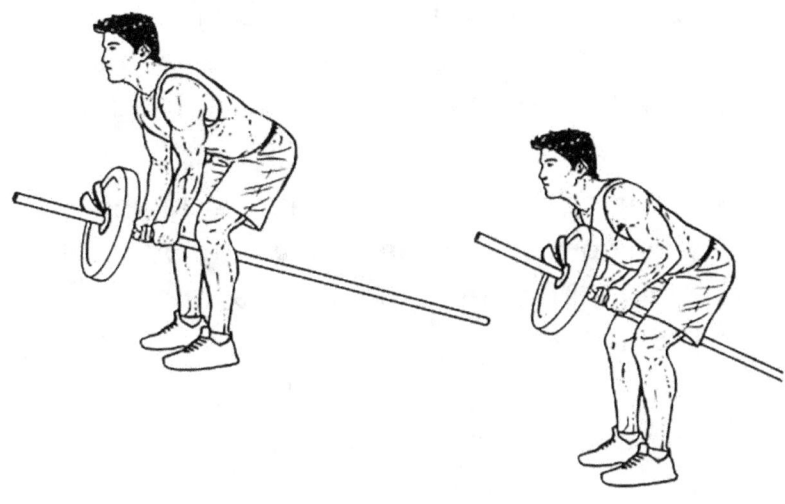

- Set up a long barbell with weight plates on one end only.

- Put the other end of the bar against a wall or something heavy so it can't slide backwards.

- Stand with one leg on either side of the bar with your knees slightly bent.

Uncommon but Effective Workouts

- Bend forward at the waist until your torso is nearly parallel to the floor.

- Grip the bar close to the weight plates with both hands, using an interlocking hands grip or neutral grip - that is one hand in front the other. This is the start position.

- Keeping your back straight in a sloping position, pull the bar straight up by bending your elbows until the plates almost touches your chest.

- Hold and squeeze your back muscles.

- Return to the start position in a slow smooth movement to place emphasis on your lats.

- Keep the bar from touching the floor.

<u>Wide Grip Seated Cable row:</u>

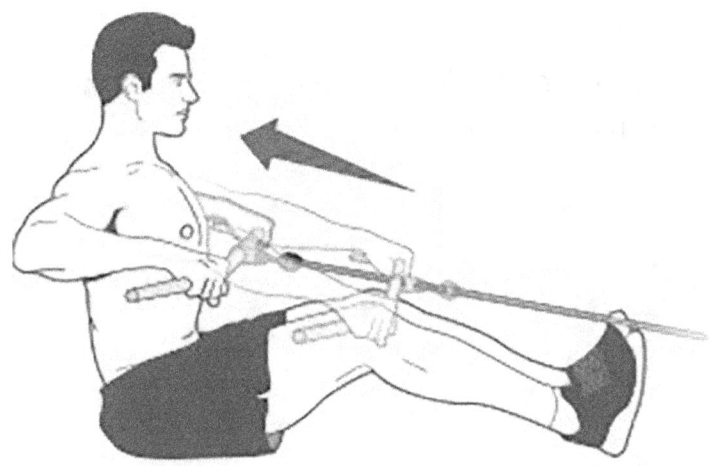

- Sit facing a low pulley machine with your legs bent comfortably and your back upright.

- Keep your chest out and shoulders back, head facing straight ahead.

- Grasp the wide-grip handle firmly and pull in towards your upper stomach, pulling your elbows as far as behind.

- Your elbows should be out wide, away from your sides. Avoid bending backward to assist with the pull.

- Only your shoulders and arms should move during this exercise.

_Variation__: Reverse grip (shoulder width) seated cable row._

Biceps Workouts:

Seated Incline bench dumbbell curl:

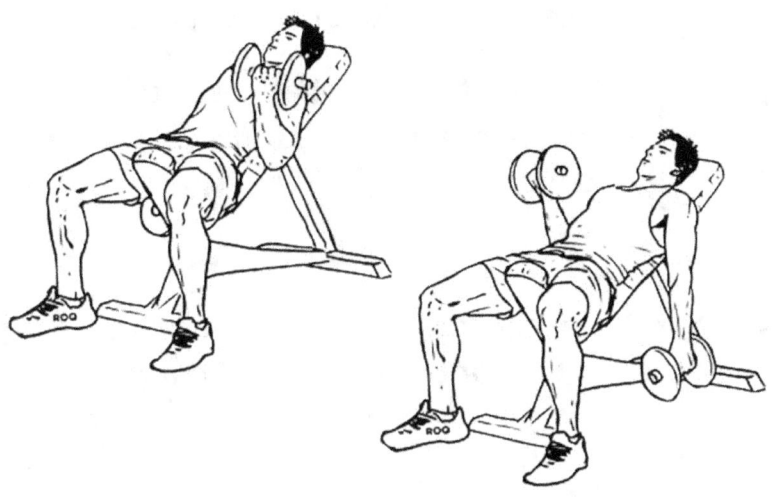

- Set up an incline bench at 45 degrees.

- Holding a dumbbell in each hand, sit on the bench, keeping your shoulders and back firmly against the back rest.

- Put your arms down by your side with your palms facing in to your body.

- Slowly curl your arms up, rotating your wrist outwards (thumbs pointing away from your body) until the dumbbell is level with your shoulders. (Your palms should be facing your shoulders)

- Flex or squeeze your bicep at the top of the movement and hold for a count of one.

- Slowly lower the dumbbells back to the start position, turning your palms back in to your body.

Variation: _You can also perform this exercise using one arm at a time or by alternating your arms_

Barbell curls lying against an Incline:

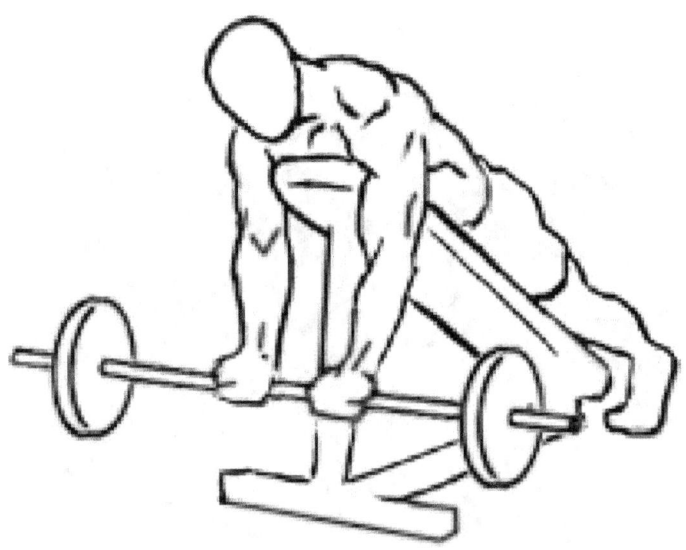

- Lay on an incline bench set up at 45 degrees with chest pressing against the bench

- Hold a barbell with shoulder width grip and rest your feet on the floor for support. And place your chin at the top of the bench comfortably.

- Hang your arms down over the bench holding onto the barbell, keeping your

elbows straight and raise the bar up
towards your head, isolating the biceps.

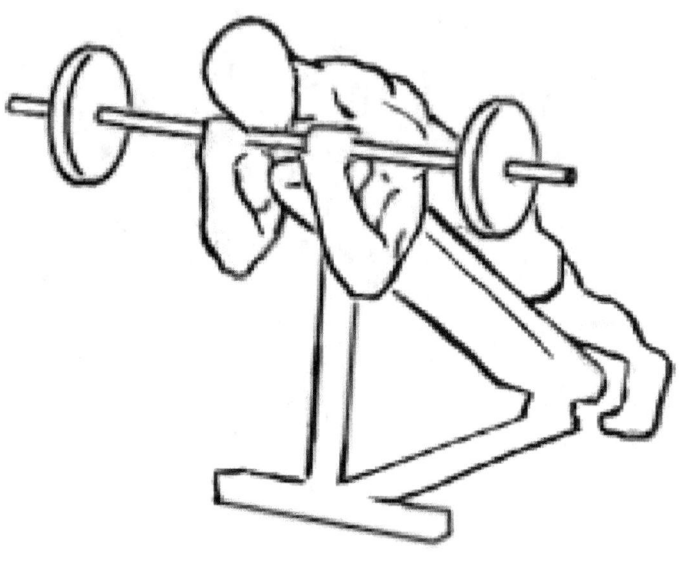

- Hold onto this position for 2 seconds then
  return back to the starting position.

Variations: _You can perform this exercise using EZ
curl bar, dumbbells and also by alternating arms._

Preacher Curl:

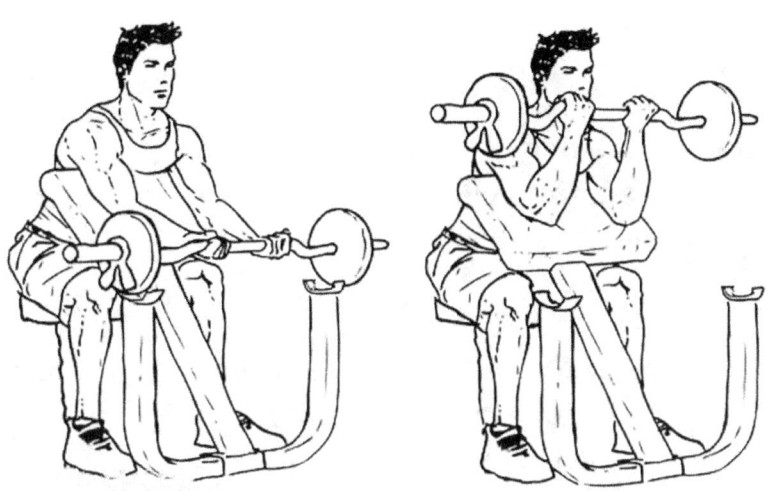

- Set up a preacher curl bench making sure that the seat is set at the right height for you. The seat shouldn't be so low that you need to raise your shoulders, or so high that you need to lean over the support pad.

- Rest your arms on the support pad with your triceps near the top and your elbows midway down the pad.

- Grip the EZ curl bar with an underhand grip at shoulder width.

- Curl the bar in towards your chin and upper chest in a single smooth arc. Hold for a count of one.

- Move only your forearms, use your bicep strength to curl the barbell up to shoulder level.

- Lower the bar by extending your arms back until your elbows are almost straight and you feel a good stretch in the biceps.

Variations: *This exercise can also be performed with a pair of dumbbells or using one arm at a time. And you can also perform this workout using a Hammer bar, and using cable rope.*

Alternate Cross Body Hammer Curl

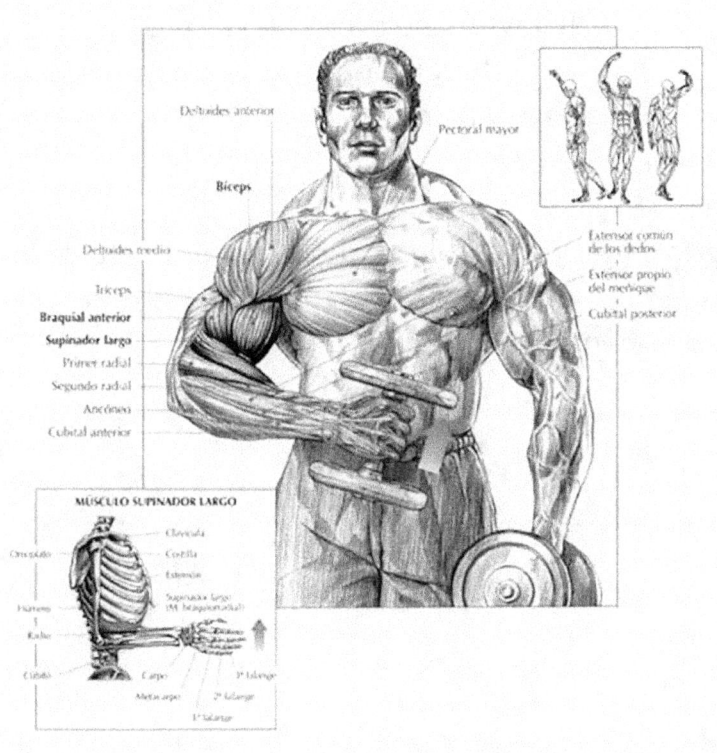

- Stand up straight with a dumbbell in each hand. Your hands should be down at your side with your palms facing in.

- While keeping your palms facing in and without twisting your arm, curl the dumbbell of the right arm up towards your left shoulder. Touch the top of the dumbbell to your shoulder and hold the contraction for a second.

- Slowly lower the dumbbell along the same path and then repeat the same movement for the left arm.

_Variations__: You can also perform this exercise in between two pulleys using the end of a rope attachment on each arm._

<u>Seated Concentration Curls</u>

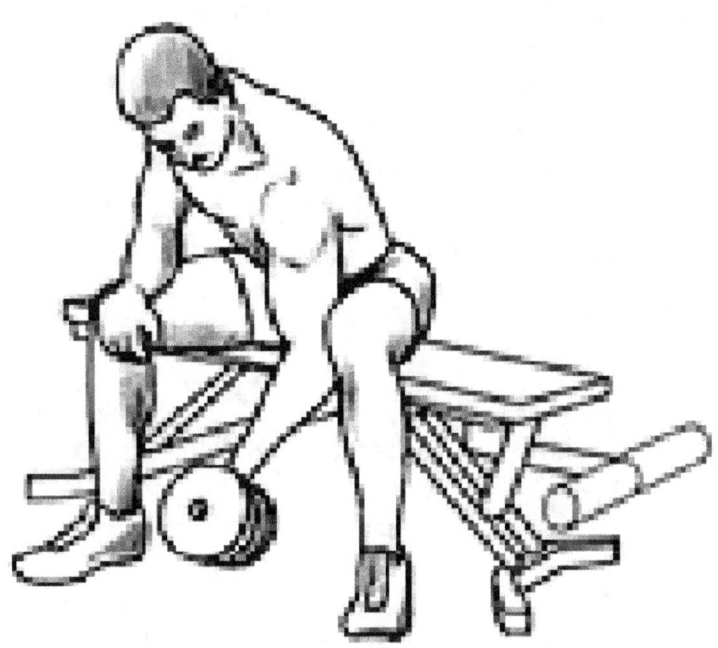

- Sit at the end of an exercise bench with your legs spread.

- Reach down between your legs and pick up a light dumbbell with one hand.

- Brace your elbow against your knee and fully straighten your arm.

- Place your other hand on your opposite leg to support your upper body.

- Moving only your forearm, use your bicep strength to curl the dumbbell up to shoulder level.

- Hold this position for a couple of seconds to maximize the peak contraction in the biceps.

- Slowly lower the dumbbell to the starting position.

- Do the same for your other arm.

Hammer curls with rope:

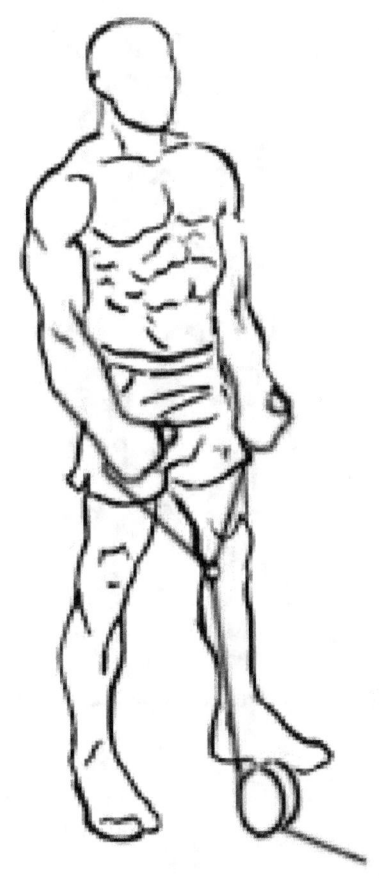

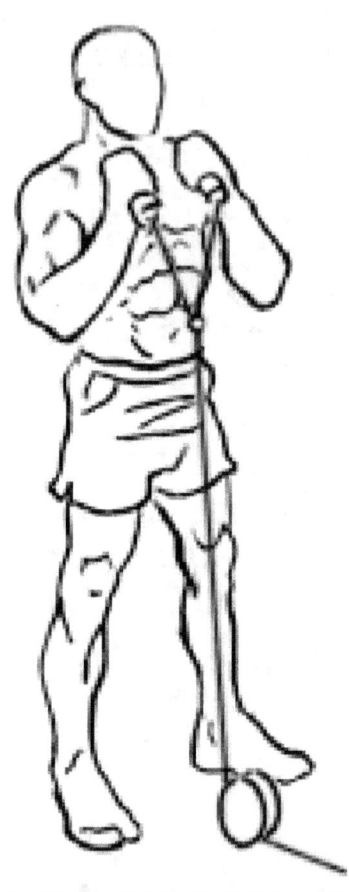

Close Grip Standing Bicep Curls

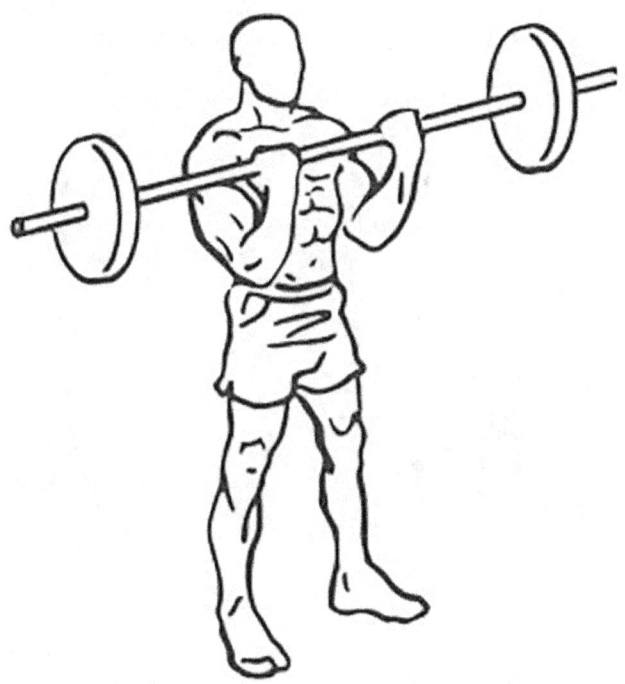

Variations:

Shoulder width grip standing bicep curl using long & heavy squat barbell.

Triceps Workouts

Bent over cable extension and Triceps Pushdown using Rope:

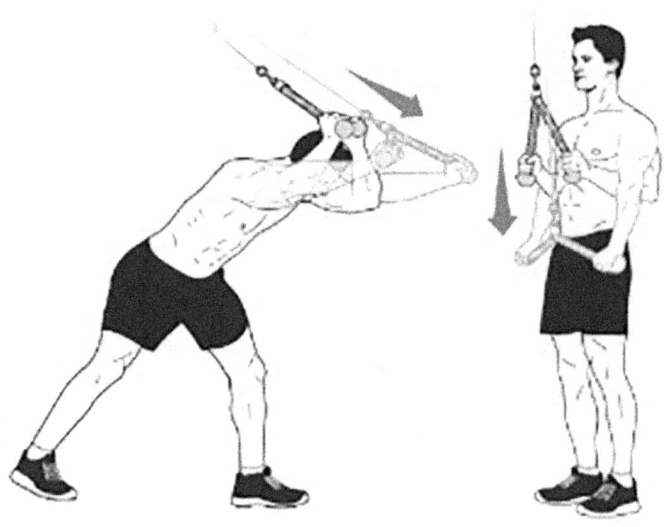

- Attach a rope to the high pulley and face away from it.

- Grab an end of the rope in each hand and bend over.

- Without moving your upper arms, push your forearms forward, pause, and return.

Triceps push down:

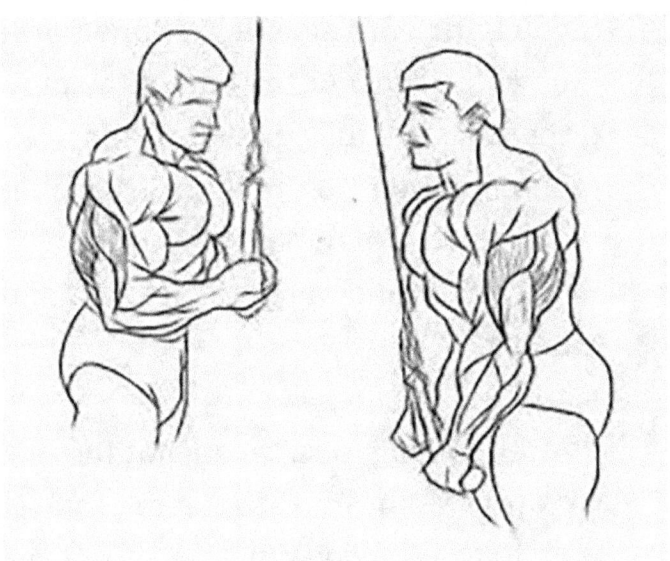

- Attach a rope attachment to a high pulley and grab with a neutral grip (palms facing each other).

- Standing upright with the torso straight and a very small inclination forward, bring the upper arms close to your body and perpendicular to the floor. The forearms should be pointing up towards the pulley as they hold the rope with the palms facing each other. This is your starting position.

- Using the triceps, bring the rope down as you bring each side of the rope to the side of your thighs. At the end of the movement the arms are fully extended and perpendicular to the floor. The upper arms should always remain stationary next to your torso and only the forearms should move.

- After holding for a second, at the contracted position, bring the rope slowly up to the starting point.

Variations: *There are many variations to this movement. For instance you can use a small bar attachment as well as a V-angled bar or straight bar.*

<u>Barbell Incline Triceps Extension:</u>

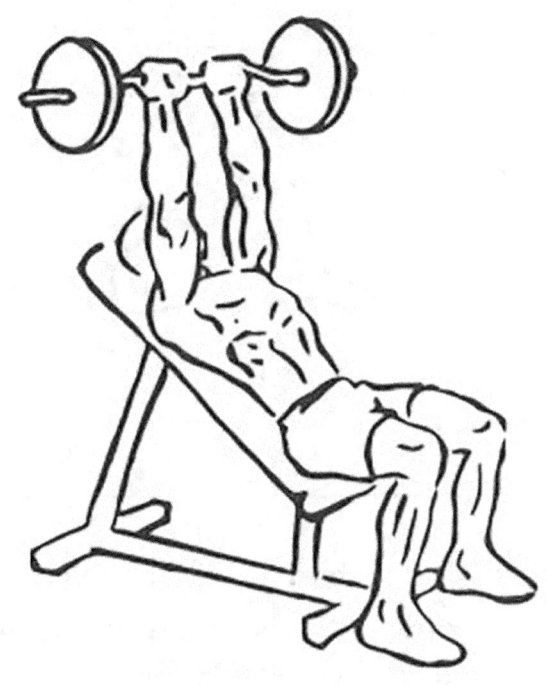

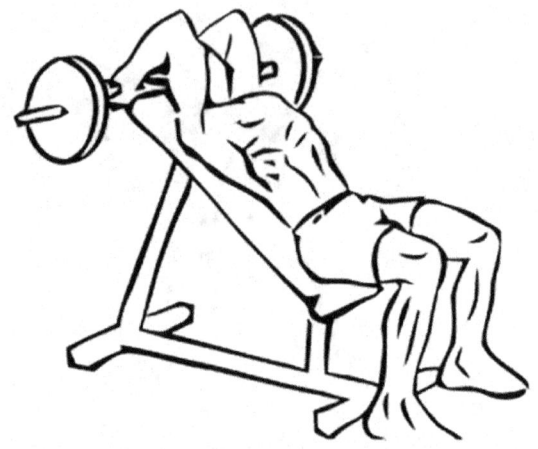

- Hold a barbell with an overhand grip (palms down) that is a little closer together than shoulder width.

- Lie back on an incline bench set at any angle between 45-75-degrees.

- Bring the bar overhead with your arms extended and elbows in. The arms should be in line with the torso above the head. This will be your starting position.

- Now lower the bar in a semicircular motion behind your head until your forearms touch your biceps. Inhale as you perform this movement. **Tip:** Keep your upper arms stationary and close to your head at all times. Only the forearms should move.

- Return to the starting position and you contract the triceps. Hold the contraction for a second.

Variations:
Can also be done with an e-z bar, with two dumbbells (using a pronated or supinated grip), seated or standing or with two dumbbells and your palms facing in.

19 SEATED EZ-BAR TRICEPS EXTENSIONS

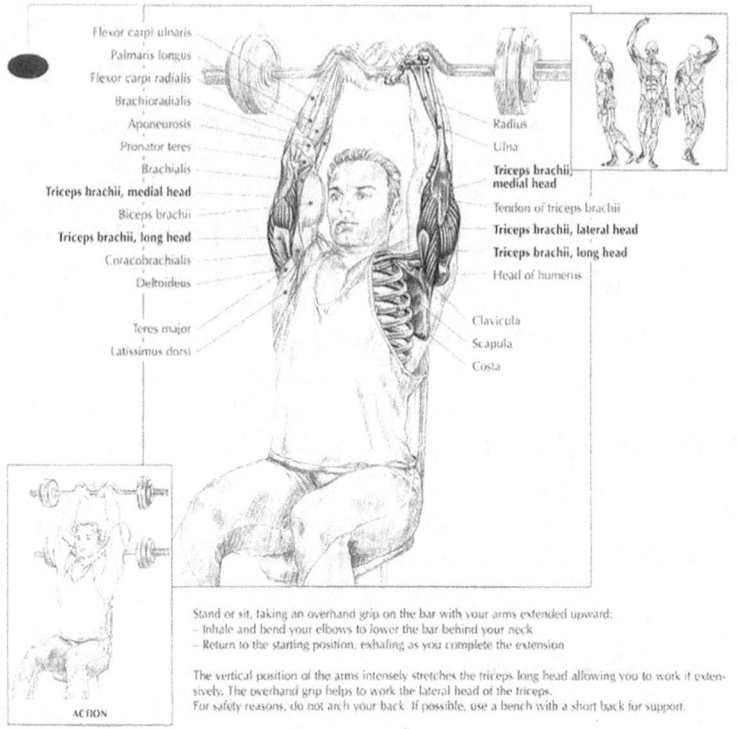

Flexor carpi ulnaris
Palmaris longus
Flexor carpi radialis
Brachioradialis
Aponeurosis
Pronator teres
Brachialis
Triceps brachii, medial head
Biceps brachii
Triceps brachii, long head
Coracobrachialis
Deltoideus
Teres major
Latissimus dorsi

Radius
Ulna
Triceps brachii, medial head
Tendon of triceps brachii
Triceps brachii, lateral head
Triceps brachii, long head
Head of humerus
Clavicula
Scapula
Costa

ACTION

Stand or sit, taking an overhand grip on the bar with your arms extended upward:
- Inhale and bend your elbows to lower the bar behind your neck
- Return to the starting position, exhaling as you complete the extension

The vertical position of the arms intensely stretches the triceps long head allowing you to work it extensively. The overhand grip helps to work the lateral head of the triceps.
For safety reasons, do not arch your back. If possible, use a bench with a short back for support.

- Stand or sit, taking an overhand grip on the bar with your arms extended upward.

- Bend your elbows to lower the bar behind your neck

- Return to the starting position

Note: The vertical position of the arms intensely stretches the triceps long head allowing you to work it extensively. The overhand grip helps to work the lateral head of the triceps.

Variations: *You can perform this workout using Dumbbells in both arms and also alternating arms.*

Reverse grip triceps extension using flat bar:

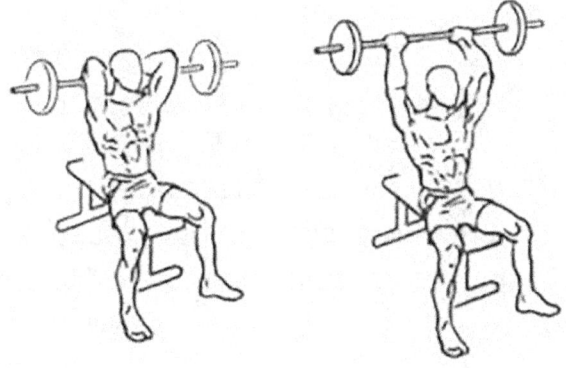

Lying Triceps Press:

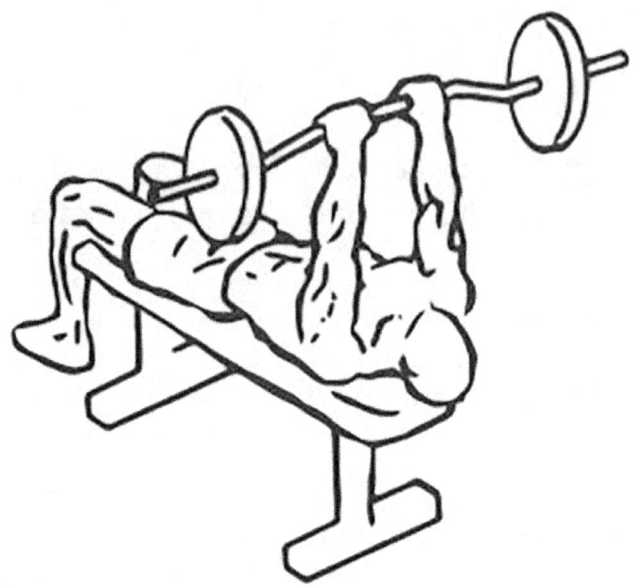

- Lie on a flat bench with either an e-z bar (my preference) or a straight bar placed on the floor behind your head and your feet on the floor.

- Grab the bar behind you, using a medium overhand (pronated) grip, and raise the bar in front of you at arm's length. **Tip:** The arms should be perpendicular to the torso and the floor. The elbows should be tucked in. This is the starting position.

- Slowly lower the weight until the bar almost touches your forehead while keeping the upper arms and elbows stationary.

- At that point, use the triceps to bring the weight back up to the starting position.

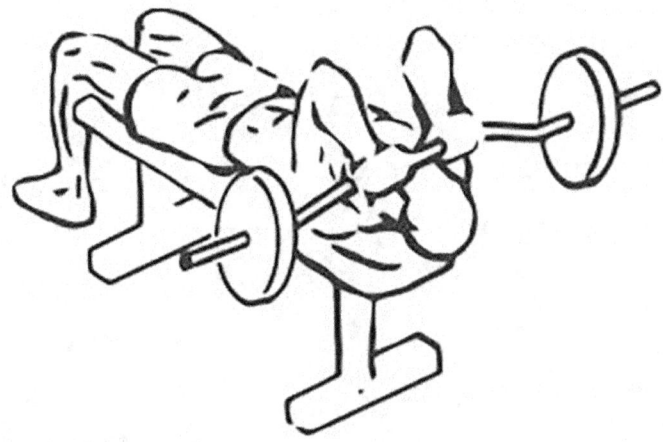

Variations:

- *There are a few variations of this exercise. You can perform it on a decline bench as opposed to a flat bench.*

- *You can also perform it using dumbbells in which case the palms of the hands will be facing each other as opposed to facing forward.*

- Also, you can try to do it using a revere grip (palms facing you).

<u>Seated dumbbell overhead triceps extension:</u>

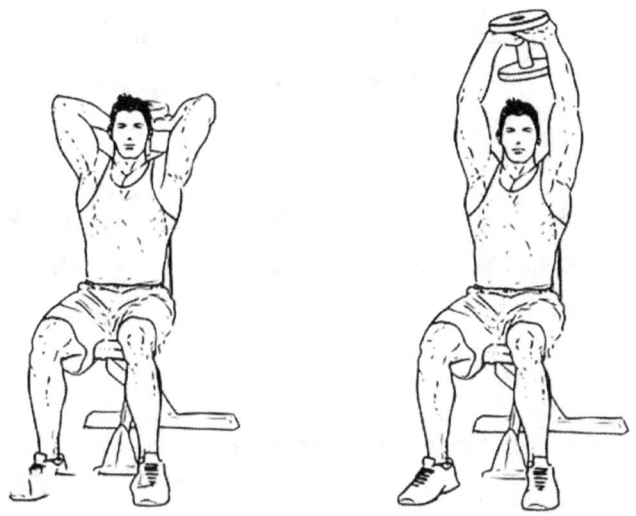

- Sit on a bench with back support.

- Grip a dumbbell at one end using both hands. Your palms should be facing inward.

- Hold the dumbbell overhead with your arms fully extended. This is the start position.

- Keep your upper arms close to your head (biceps roughly level with your temples) and near to 90degrees to the floor.

- Moving only your forearms, lower the dumbbell in a smooth arc behind your head until your forearms and biceps touch. Hold for a count of one.

- Return to the start position by using the triceps to extend your arm and raise the dumbbell.

Note: *This exercise can be performed standing. However, it places an extra strain on your back.*

Variations: *You can also perform this exercise using an EZ bar or straight bar with a close grip behind your head, palms facing forward.*

SEATED DUMBBELL TRICEPS EXTENSIONS 18

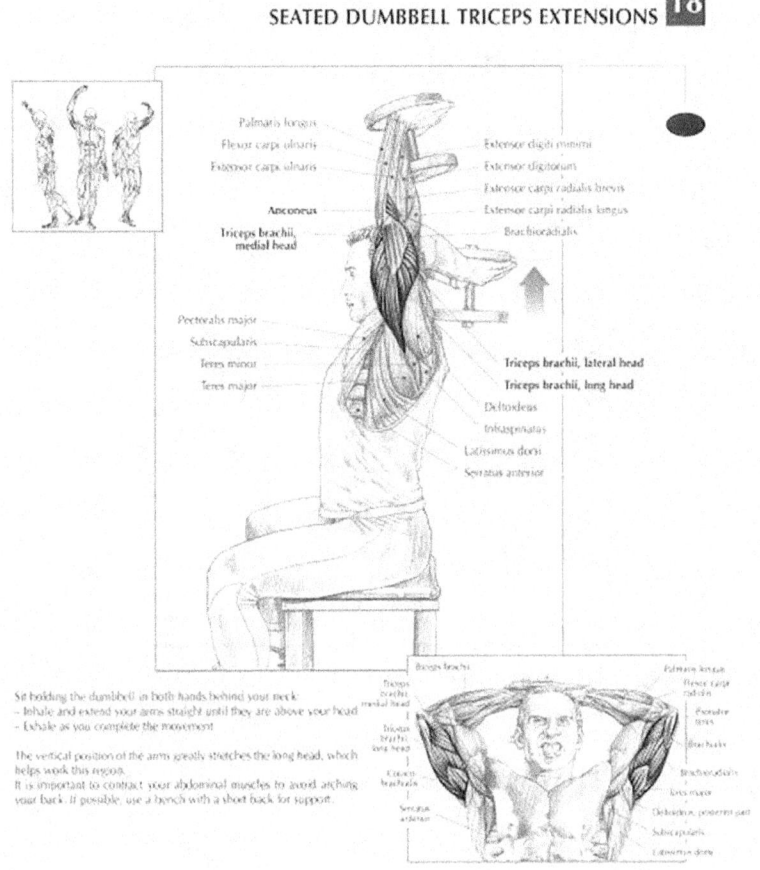

Sit holding the dumbbell in both hands behind your neck
– Inhale and extend your arms straight until they are above your head
– Exhale as you complete the movement

The vertical position of the arm greatly stretches the long head, which
helps work this region.
It is important to contract your abdominal muscles to avoid arching
your back. If possible, use a bench with a short back for support.

Sit holding the dumbbell in both hands behind
your neck and extend your arms straight until they
are above your head as you complete the
movement.

<u>One arm triceps extension:</u>

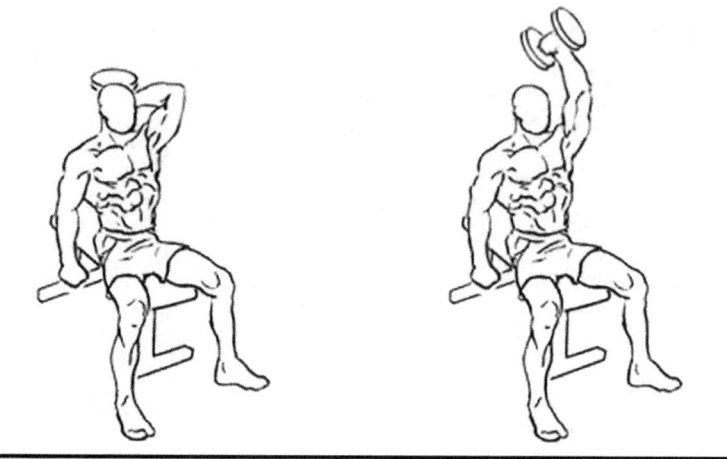

- Sit on a bench or chair. Hold a dumbbell in one hand.

- Extend your arms so the weight is over your head (biceps roughly level with your temples) and near to 90degrees to the floor.

- Keeping your upper arm and elbow stationary and close to your head, lower the dumbbell in an arc behind your head.

- Feel the triceps stretch as far as possible and then press the dumbbell back up to the starting position.

- Finish your set working one arm only and then repeat the movement with the other arm.

Parallel bar dips:

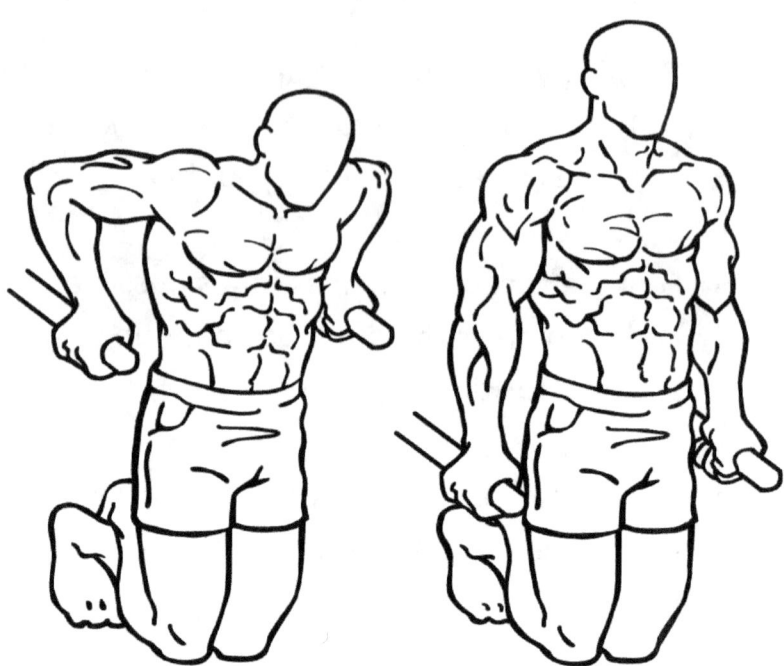

- Support yourself with your arms straight and your torso hanging down from your shoulders

- Bend your elbows to allow your body to sink as far as down between the bars as possible.

- Reverse the motion and return to the starting point.

Bench triceps dips:

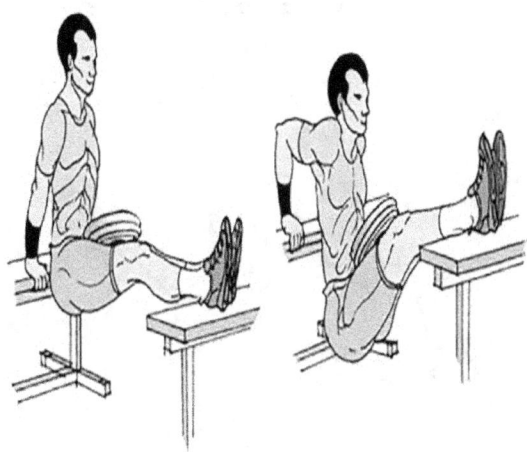

- Place your hands on the edge of a flat bench and rest your feet on another bench. Assume a torso-leg angle at about a 90 degree

- Bend your elbows to allow your body sink as far as down between the benches as possible.

- Straighten your arms to return to the starting position.

  Note : *For more workout intensify, you can place a weight on your thighs.*

Chest Workouts:

Dumbbell Bench Press:

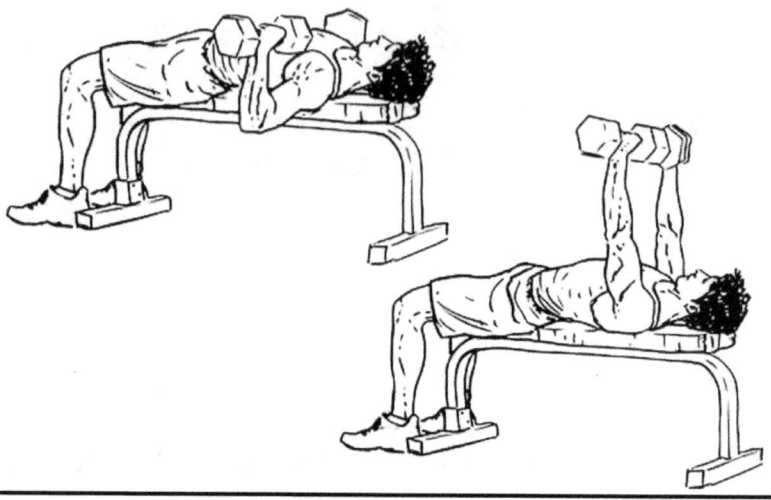

- Lie on a flat bench holding a dumbbell in each hand with an overhand grip.

- Start by holding the dumbbells slightly wider than shoulder width apart above your shoulders. Your palms should be facing forward.

- Slowly bend your elbows until they are at a 90 degree angle and your upper arms are parallel to the ground.

- Push the weights up by straightening your arms.

- As you push the weights up, move your arms in an arc to bring the dumbbells together, until they meet over the center of your chest. Hold for a count of one.

- Lower the dumbbells by slowly bending your elbows back to 90 degrees.

- Continue lowering your arms until they are a little lower than parallel to the floor. (Your elbows should be pointing slightly towards the floor and you should feel a stretch in your chest muscles and shoulders.)

  Note: _Be sure to concentrate on a balanced movement when lifting the dumbbells. Use both arms equally spaced and moving at the same speed._

Incline Dumbbell Fly

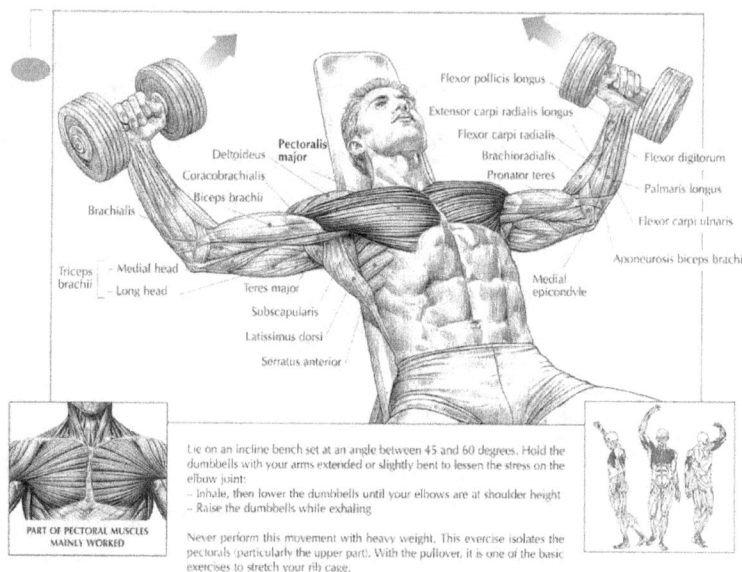

INCLINE DUMBBELL FLYS

Lie on an incline bench set at an angle between 45 and 60 degrees. Hold the dumbbells with your arms extended or slightly bent to lessen the stress on the elbow joint:
– Inhale, then lower the dumbbells until your elbows are at shoulder height
– Raise the dumbbells while exhaling

Never perform this movement with heavy weight. This exercise isolates the pectorals (particularly the upper part). With the pullover, it is one of the basic exercises to stretch your rib cage.

- Set up an incline bench at about 30 degrees.

- Lie on the bench and hold a dumbbell in each hand with an overhand grip.

- Make sure you keep your back flat and your shoulders pushed back

- Turn your hands in so that your palms are facing each other, holding the dumbbells over your chest with your elbows slightly bent and pointing outwards.

- Lower the dumbbells out to the side of your shoulders, while keeping your elbows slightly bent in a smooth arcing motion.

- Continue lowering them until you feel a stretch in your chest and shoulders. Pause for a count of one.

- Bring the dumbbells back to the starting position in the same smooth arc with your elbows slightly bent until the dumbbells are nearly touching.

Note: Don't perform this exercise with heavy weight. This exercise isolates the pectorals (particularly the upper part). With the "dumbbell pullover", it is one of the effective exercises to stretch your rib cage.

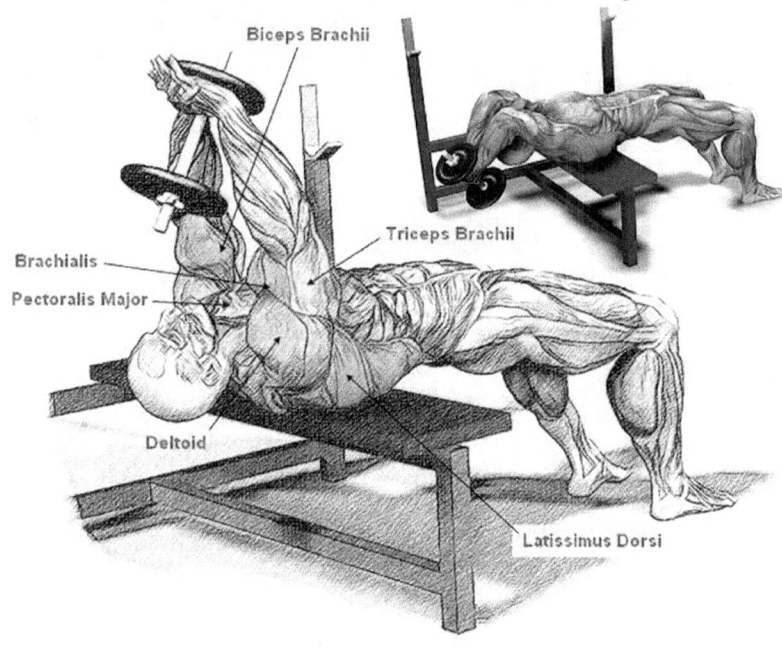

Dumbell Pullover Anatomy

Cable Crossover:

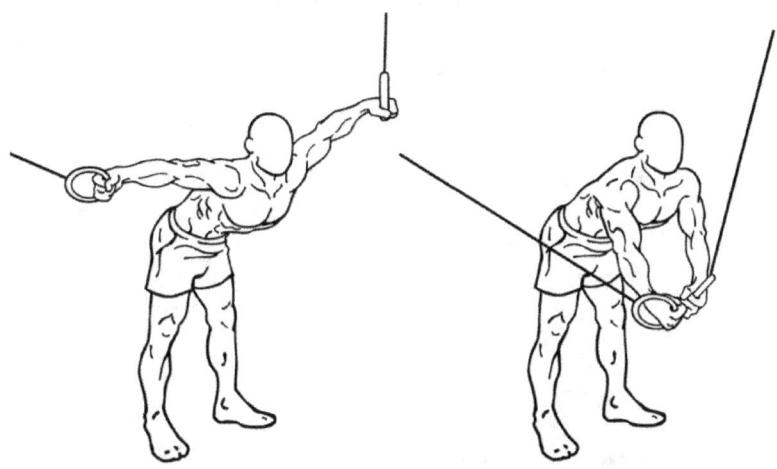

- Set up the pulley with the handles at shoulder height

- Stand a foot in front of the machine with one foot in front of the other

- Slightly bend forward at waist for good balance and grip the handles. This is your starting position

- Bring your hands together in front of your chest, maintaining a slight bend in the elbows.
- Pause at the bottom of the movement, squeezing the pecs together, before slowly returning to the start position

Close grip bench press:

Close Grip Bench Press (start)

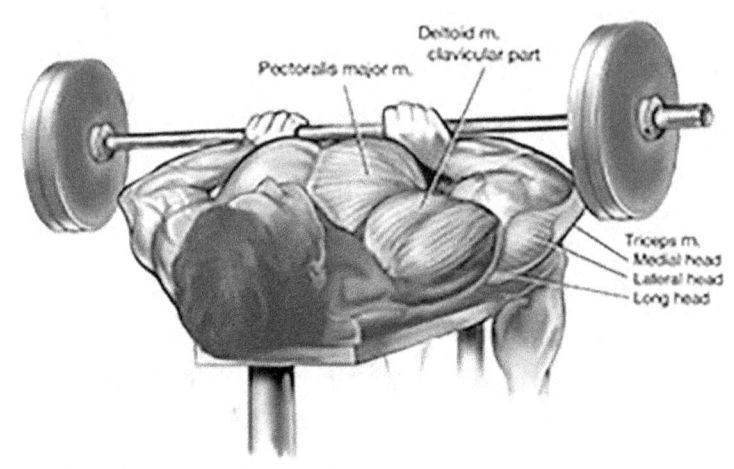

- Set up on a flat bench with your feet planted firmly on the floor

- Grip the bar just inside shoulder width

- Raise the bar so it's above the middle of your chest

- Slowly lower the bar until it's just above your chest, then push it back to the starting position

- When you reach the top of the movement, squeeze your pecs together

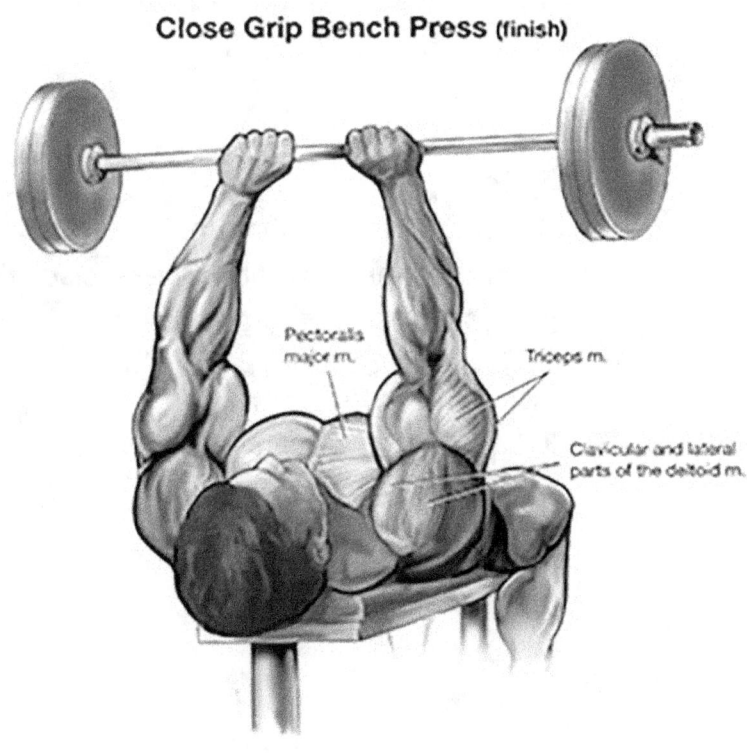

Close Grip Bench Press (finish)

Uncommon but Effective Workouts

Regular Chest Workouts:

I) Flat Bench Press with Barbell, Smith Machine and Dumbbells

II) Inclined Bench press with Barbell, Smith Machine and Dumbbells

III) Declined Bench press with Barbell, Smith Machine and Dumbbells

Note: By alternating between Barbell, Dumbbell, Hydraulic machines/Cable machines, and Free hand exercises like pullups, pushups, dips etc.),you can get variety on your workouts thereby keeping monotony at bay, as well as increase momentum on your strength and development. This logic applies for all workouts.

Legs Workouts:

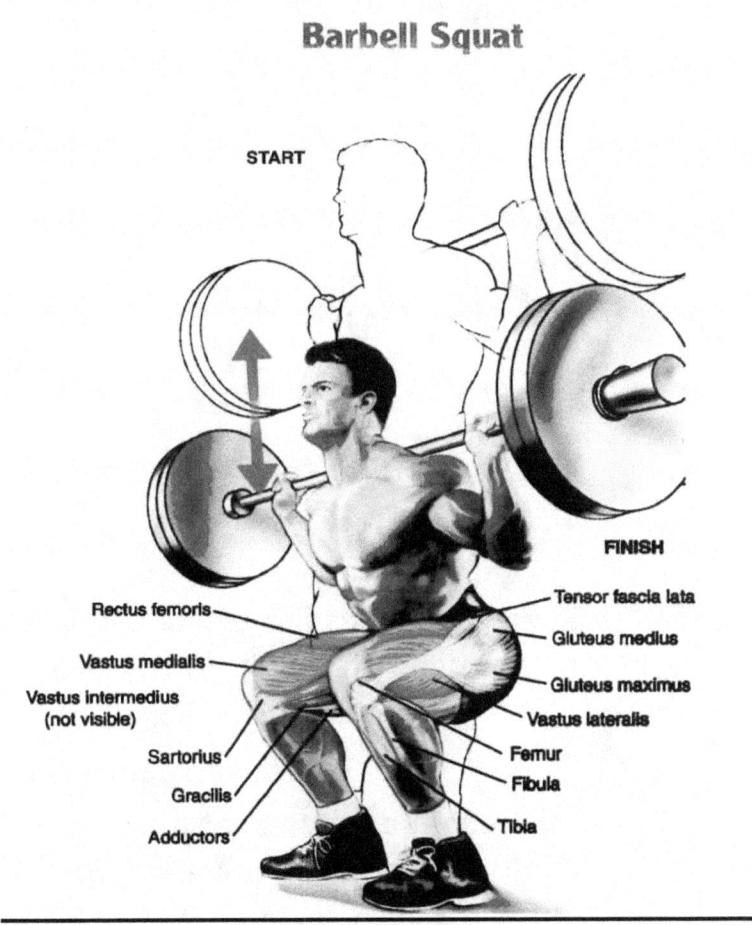

Barbell Squat

- Set up the barbell on the squat rack so that it is at the same height as your upper chest.

Uncommon but Effective Workouts

- Position your body under the bar, with knees bent so that the bar is resting high on the back of your shoulders.

- Grip the bar with your hands comfortably wider than your shoulders.

- Slowly straighten your legs to push upwards, lifting the barbell from the rack and take one step forward.

- Stand with your legs shoulder width apart.

- Bend your knees forward and allow your hips to bend back as if sitting down.

- Continue this movement down until your thighs are parallel to the floor or slightly more, making sure your knees are pointing in the same direction as your feet.

- Hold for a count of one.

- Push up through your heels while straightening your hips and knees, until you are standing in the start position.

- Make any adjustments necessary to your stance and grip before continuing on the next repetition.

  Notes: _Do not rest the bar on your neck. Keep your head facing forward at all times. Keep your back straight throughout the entire movement._

  Variation:
  Another effective variant of squat is Machine Hack Squat.

  You can also perform squat using, Smith Machine.

Leg Press:

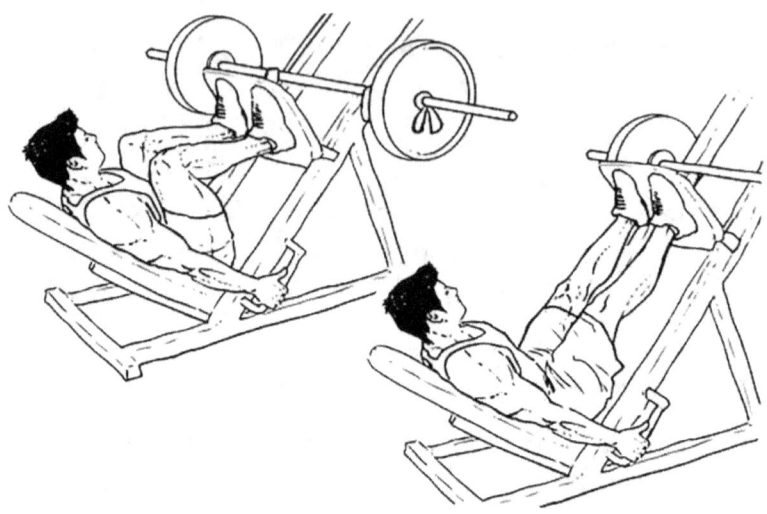

- Sit down on a leg press machine and place your legs on the platform directly in front of you at shoulder width.

- Lower the safety bars holding the weighted platform and press the platform all the way up until your legs are fully extended in front of you bot *do NOT* lock your knees. Your torso and legs should be at a 90degree angle to each other. This is the start position.

- Slowly lower the platform until your upper and lower legs form a 90-degree angle. Pause for a count of one.

- Return to the starting position by pushing through the heels of your feet, engaging your quadriceps.

__Variation__: You can perform this workout by alternating legs. That is using one leg at a time to press. But make sure to use comfortable weights, don't use heavy weights. Also support your knees with hands, thereby making sure the workout is felt only on your thigs and not on your knees.

Seated Machine Leg Extensions:

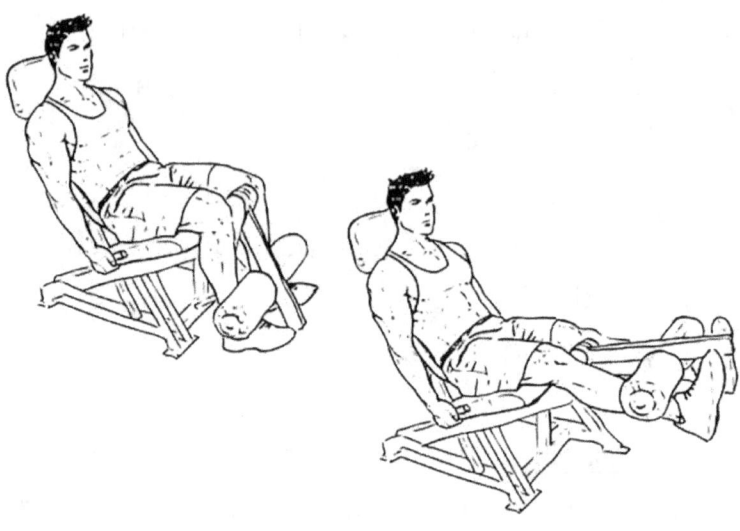

- Sit on a leg extension machine and place your legs under the pad with your feet pointed forward. The pad should rest on your shins just above your feet and you will need to adjust it to suit.

- Grip the hand bars (if fitted) firmly. This is the start position.

- Using only your quadriceps, fully extend your legs exhaling as you do so. Hold for a count of one.

- Return to the start position in a smooth movement as you inhale.

- The angle at your knee should not go past 90-degrees.

Variation: *This exercise can be performed one leg at a time.*

Lying Leg Curls:

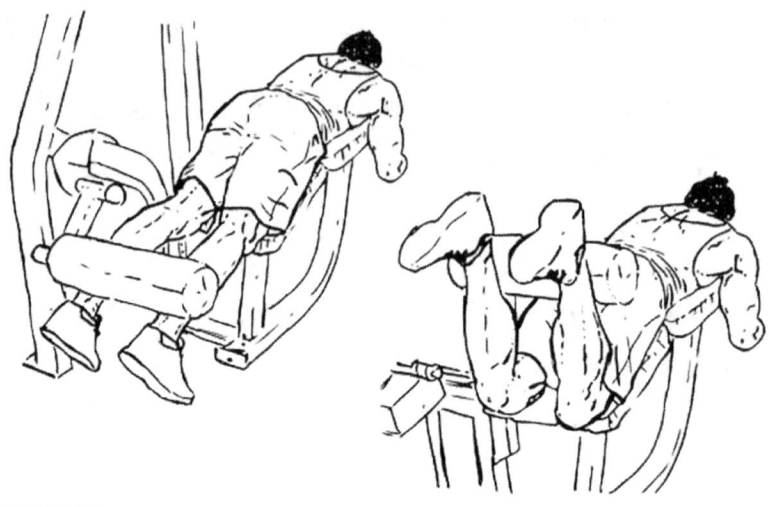

- Lie face down on a leg curl machine and lock your heels under the foot pad. Make sure your legs are fully extended and the foot pads are resting on the back of your ankles.

- If the machine is equipped with handles, grip them. If not, grip the front of the pad you are lying on.
- Remaining flat on the bench, with no arching of your spine, curl your legs up in a smooth arcing motion by bending your knees until your hamstrings are fully contracted. Hold for a count of one.

- Slowly lower your legs to the starting position in a smooth arcing motion.

Variation: *This exercise can be performed one leg at a time.*

<u>Jump Squat:</u>

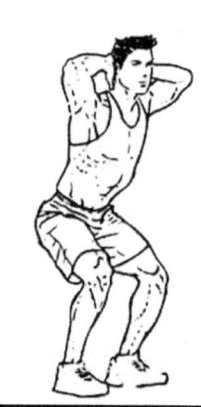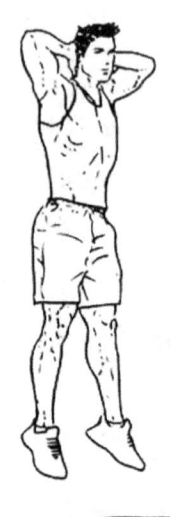

- Stand with your feet hip width apart. Your toes should be pointing straight ahead or only slightly outward.

- Cross your arms in front of your body, place your hands behind your head or at the sides of your head.

- Keep your weight on your heels and bend your knees while lowering your hips towards the ground as if you are sitting down on a chair.

- Keep your back straight at all times.

- Continue until you feel a slight stretch in your quadriceps. Do not let your knees extend out beyond the level of your toes.

- Pause for a count of one.

- In an explosive movement, drive down through your heels pushing yourself up of the floor with your quads.

- At the same time extend our arms out above you.

- Land with your knees slightly bent to absorb the impact.

Inner Thighs / Abductor-Adductor machine:

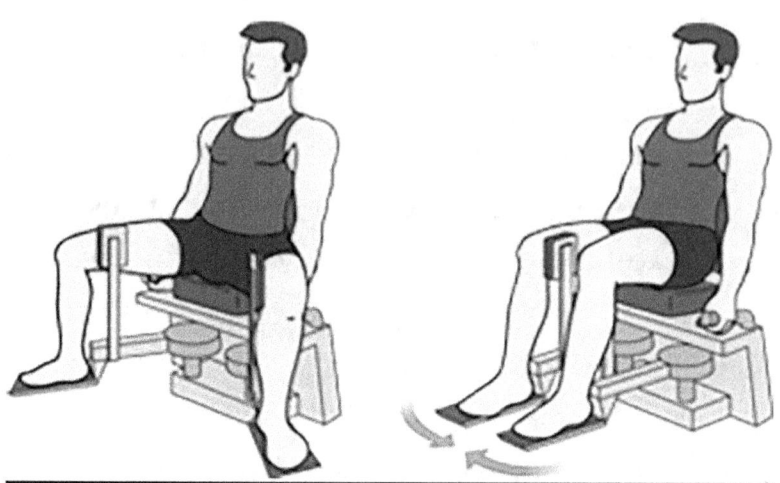

- Set up an abductor machine by selecting and appropriate weight and adjusting the seat and leg pads to a comfortable position.

- If fitted, grasp the handles on each side of the machine.

- Keep your entire upper body straight and stationary with your back pressed firmly against the back rest. This is the start position.

Uncommon but Effective Workouts

- Press against the legs pads of the machine with your legs, by slowly spreading them.

- When you feel a slight stretching in your abductors, pause fora count of one squeezing them as you do so.

- In a controlled movement, return to the start position.

  __Variation:__ Place your thigs inside the abductor machine and stretch your legs outwards. Just reverse of previous movement.

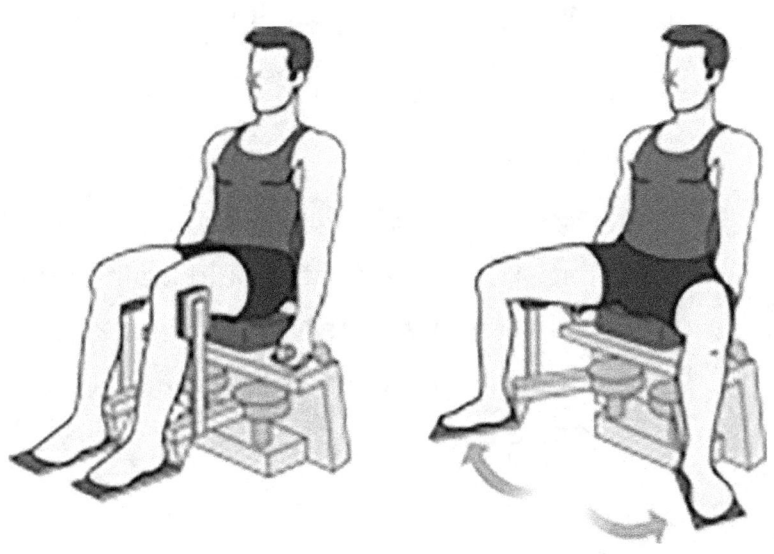

Dumbbell Lunges:

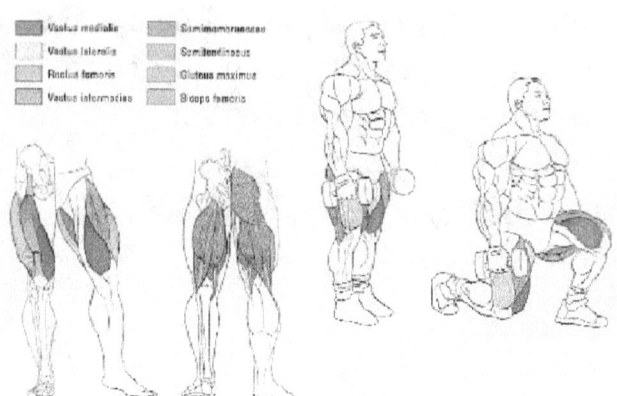

1. Holding a dumbbell in each hand, stand with your feet shoulder width apart.

2. Keep your shoulders back. And your back straight.

3. Take a long stride forward with your right leg. Your right foot should be in a position, that when you bend your right knee, your upper and lower leg forms a 90 degree angle.

4. Slowly bend both your knees, to lower your hips until your left (rear) knee is just above the floor. Hold for a count of one.

5. Return to the start position by slowly straightening your legs and raising your body back to a standing position.

6. Complete all the repetitions for one set full set, then switch legs, or you can alternate between legs for each rep.

Note: *Do not let your knee travel past your toes in the down position as this can cause instability and injury.*

How to strategically use Swimming:

Swimming is a high-end full-body workout that increases your aerobic potential and also offers resistance. This activity engages nearly every muscle in the body. It improves blood circulation which helps to scrape away the small layers of cholesterol or other toxins within the blood vessels.

Swimming Improves Flexibility, Posture & Balance:

Flexibility refers to our range of motion. This includes the ability to maneuver our hands, feet, neck and the back. Swimming is a rare exercise since apart from working the muscles; it also stretches the muscle fibers and ligaments. This is vital for maintaining the tension in our tendons that supports various bodily movements. People often suffer from musculoskeletal problems due to bad posture or loss of muscle tone. Swimming is the only low-impact exercise that requires the entire body to function coherently. This means it forces the body to realign itself in a more uniform manner. This is vital for completing those laps around the swimming pool. This is how swimming gifts us with better balance and posture.

Swimming is a Great Stress Buster:

Swimming is a great way to burn-away the blues. The act of plunging into a pool and splashing through water tends to engage our body and mind. This takes away our preoccupation with any troubling thought. Being a full-body exercise, swimming has the effects of a high-impact workout at the gym. This induces the release of endorphins. These are the body's feel-good hormones that help to neutralize that depressive feeling. Further, the buoyant action of the water has a massage-like effect on the body, helping us to relax.

Swimming Increases Muscular Strength & Aids Overall Physical Conditioning:

Swimming is a unique exercise since it works the core muscles apart from the upper and lower limb simultaneously. It helps in increasing our overall physical conditioning. Swimming tends work the joints without inducing the risk of an injury. Please note that there is a difference between becoming powerful and having bigger biceps. Curling weights in the gym can get you bigger muscles but swimming helps you become stronger, i.e. it raises your muscular strength. Swimming comprehensively works all the bigger muscle groups like the chest, shoulder, thigh and back muscles.

Cardio-respiratory Endurance:

This means, how well your heart and lungs send blood and oxygen to the muscles that are being used.

Your cardiovascular system is always pumping oxygen and blood through your body so it keeps on working normally while you kick, breathe, and move your arms repeatedly. This cycle is completed for a timing of at least 20 minutes. The amount of oxygen needed is very high and the endurance level in your body helps you convert energy stores into fuel for your body.

Muscular Endurance:

Muscular endurance is, being able to use your muscles over and over again without getting tired.

Swimming usually demands muscular endurance in order to help your body perform a cardiorespiratory endurance motion. Your body needs certain level of strength so it can move faster and not get so tired.

Muscular Strength:

That is, how well your muscles are for a short period of time.

Water is always acting as a resistance factor against the human body and as a swimmer, the body should be able to overcome that water resistance. Muscles such as the latissimus dorsi muscle, which is the largest muscle in our back is the one that helps a swimmer move his arms in every direction through water and is also the most active muscle in all the strokes that can possibly exist. Shoulders, arms and long limbs allow the swimmer to thrust and drag.

Swimming greatly stimulates Appetite:

This is one of the most helpful aspects of swimming for skinny persons. The common suggested theory is that the pool's cooler temperature causes your body to lose heat, which can stop your body from releasing appetite-suppressing hormones.

Different Strokes of Swimming:

Different swimming strokes target different muscle groups, so for optimal benefits, vary your stroke selection. Bear in mind, that your least-favorite stroke may do you the most good.

It will work muscles that may be weaker in the body, helping you overcome muscular imbalances.

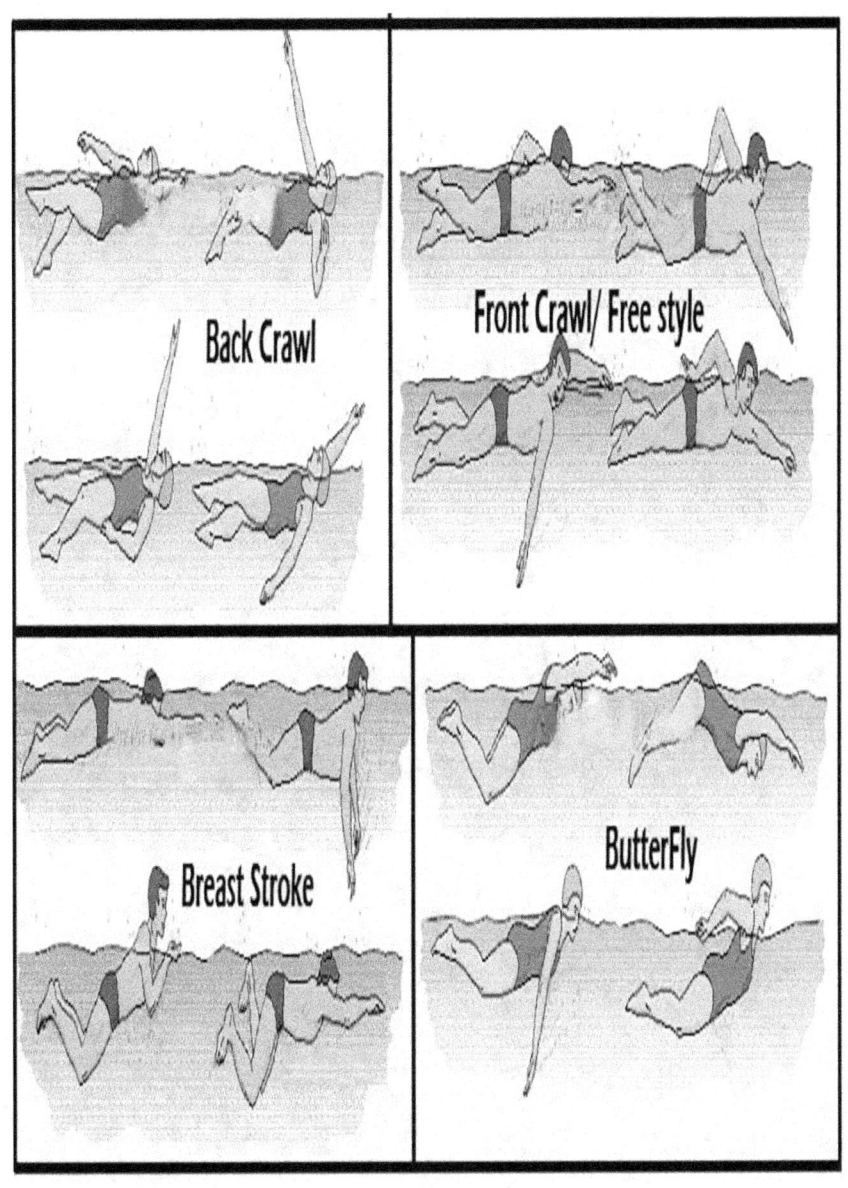

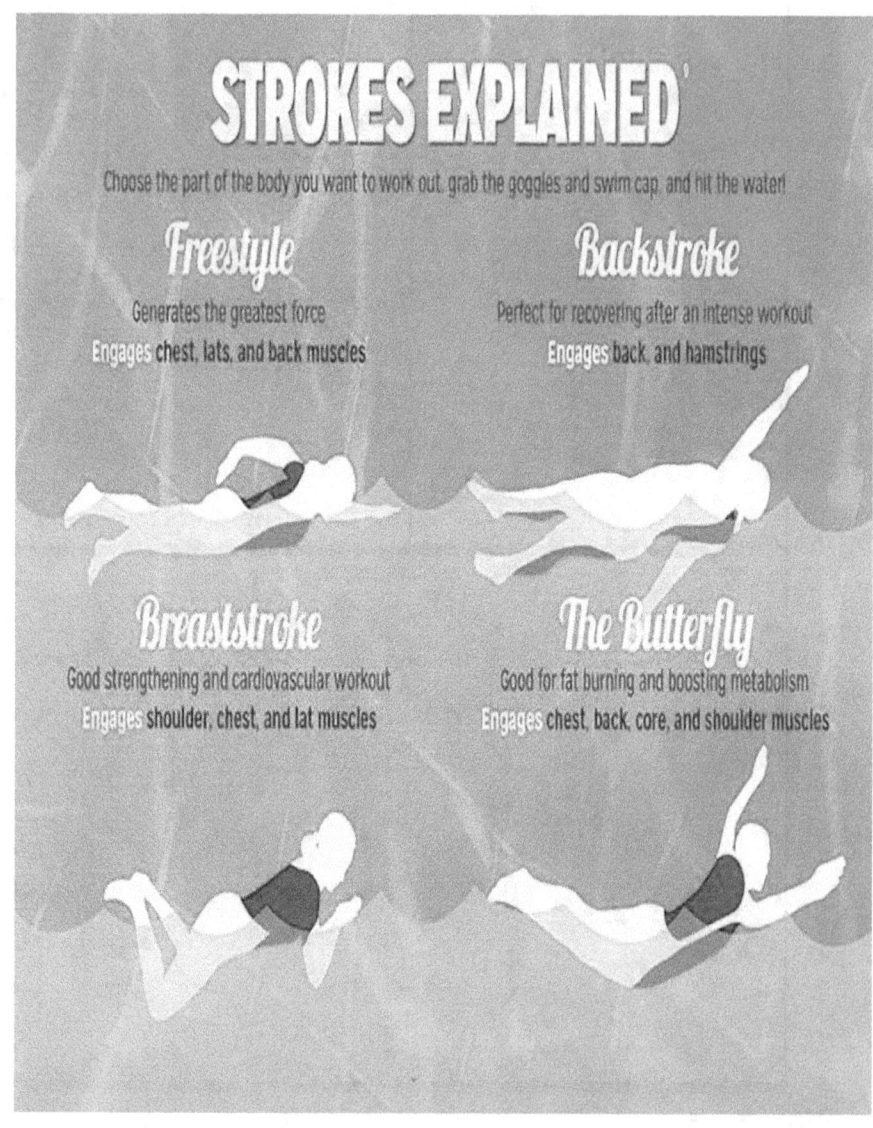

The Front Crawl:

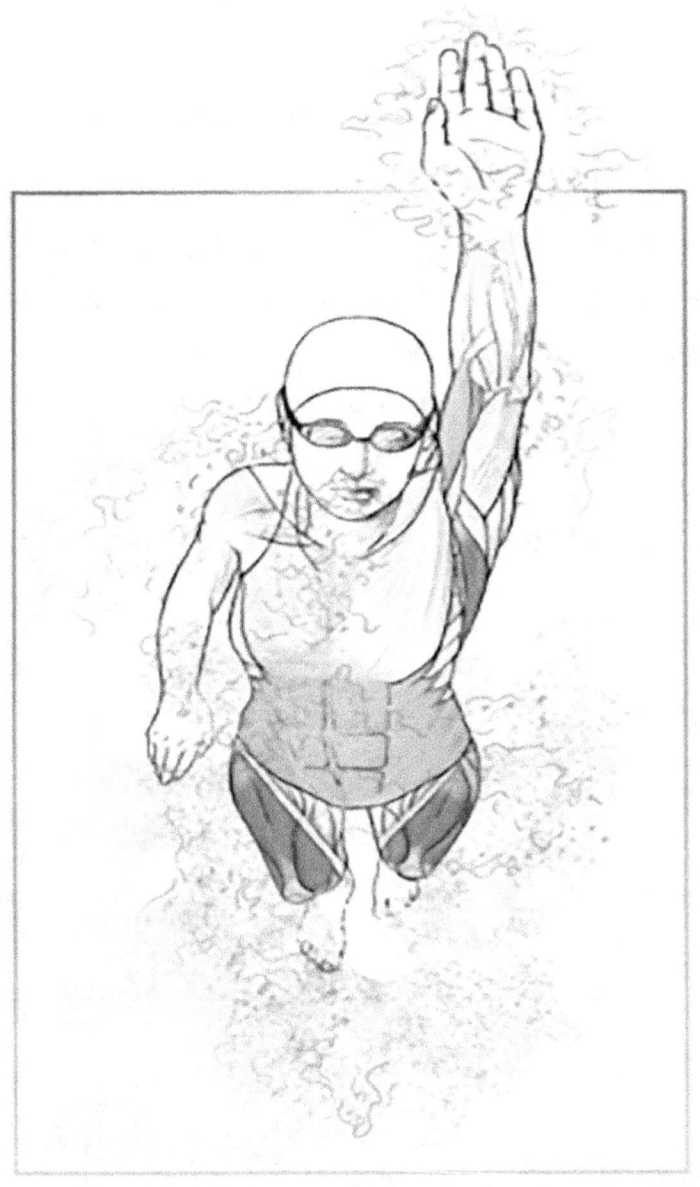

The front crawl stroke is great for those who enjoy faster paced swimming because it generates the most force.

This stroke recruits the chest muscles, the lats, and other back muscles.

Because this exercise requires rapid movement of the arms, going from above the head to down by the sides of the body, you'll tap into your fast-twitch muscle fiber potential, leading to improvements in speed and power.

The Backstroke:

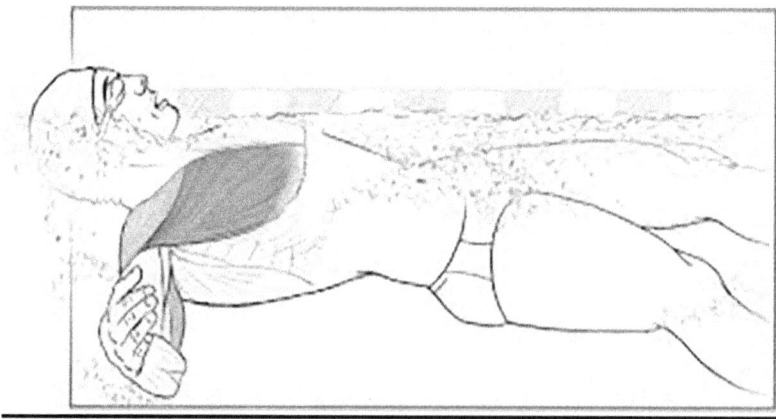

This stroke is less intensive than the front crawl or breaststroke. If you're doing a recovery swim between intense workouts at the gym, this should be your go-to stroke.

Not surprisingly, this stroke will hammer your back. Your lats pull your arms beneath the water and then back to the surface again.

Your hamstrings come into play slightly more due to the back-down position.

The Breaststroke:

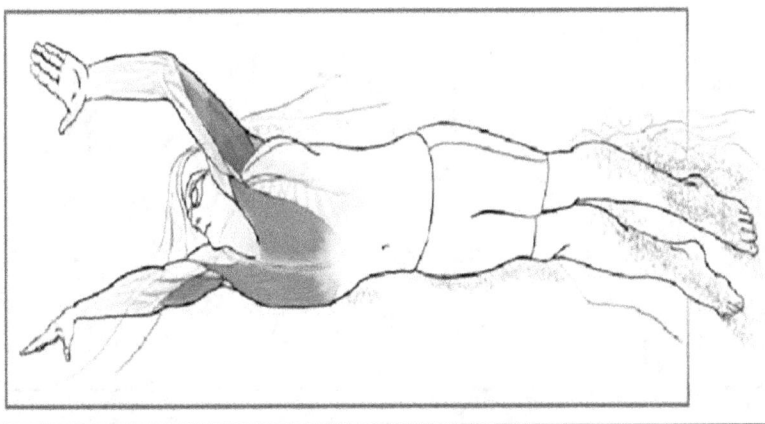

The breaststroke is one of the most popular swimming strokes and involves your lower and upper body moving in sync. The breaststroke is swum in a prone position, with both arms moving synchronously in short, half-circular movements under water. The legs also move synchronously and execute a whip kick.

The breaststroke is great for any beginner because it's easy on the body. You don't have to exert a ton of effort, so it's easier to swim several laps before getting fatigued.

The Butterfly:

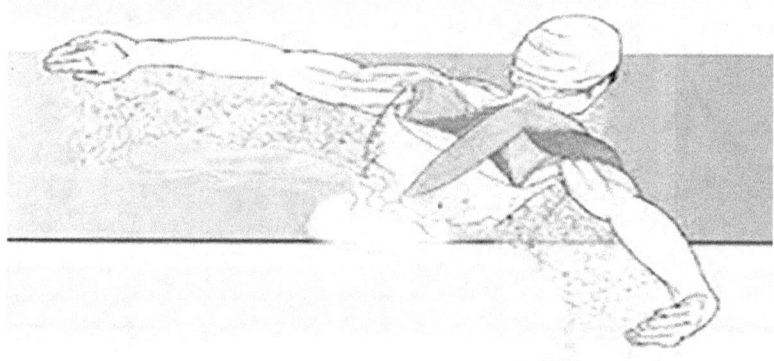

This stroke is excellent for boosting your metabolism; targeting your chest, shoulders, and back; and helping to build better power and strength.

Use Swimming Strategically

This stroke requires the arms to move forward simultaneously, then into the water and back again. Your core will scream as it keeps your body stabilized moving through the water.

This is a great stroke to perform as interval training sessions in the water. The intensity will make it easily possible.

Based on the information about different aspects of swimming provided above, it is you who need to find how to strategically utilize the positive impacts of swimming which is required for your body's transformation. You need to find areas that require improvement and scope and different means of doing it. That is you can use if for muscular endurance, recovery from weight training, massaging effects on muscles, great stress busting effects, muscle toning, great appetizing effect. As with any form of exercise, create balance in your program between swimming workouts, weight training workouts, active rest and recovery.

Sustain Transformation

There is a vital final step in the process of transformation, which comes after you got your body transformed, that is sustaining what you have achieved. The reason I stress on the importance of sustaining is because, what you had achieved is not 100% natural. In the process of transformation you have got the critical help from few performance enhancers to break the genetic shackles, which is not your body's natural process. Hence that which you got with the use of certain external factors, needs care taking/safeguarding for certain period in-order to make your gains an integral part of yourself.

This is not a difficult thing to do. What you have to do is just continue what you have been doing, for certain period of time. You will know by yourself that you have successfully sustained your gains over a period of time. Until then don't bring the process to complete halt, though you can gradually reduce the intensity of your workouts. Just remember not to bring the process to a grinding halt, immediately after the success of your mission.

Valuable Insights

> Body transformation is a chain reaction, every aspect in that chain must be in alignment/harmony to make the body machine move.

> It is most important to understand that mission transformation is a gradual process which needs more time.

> Persistent and dedicated exploration & experimentation of various physical activities with the aid of few performance enhancers will lead to body transformation.

> It is better to concentrate on doing the work-outs correctly with proper technique rather than blindly increasing weights of dumbbell/barbell for the sake of others.

> Proper resting/muscle recovery is an integral part of gaining muscles.

Valuable Insights

- ➢ Evening time workouts, 3 to 4 hours after lunch will be advantageous for building muscles, than early morning workouts on empty stomach.

- ➢ Barbell/Dumbbell workouts help in improving your muscle mass. Cable/Hydraulic machine workouts help you get in shape. Freehand workouts like pullups pushups, dips improve gaining power.

- ➢ Even minor variations in angles of bench, hand grip position, elbow position, body posture will involve different set of muscles. And this is what improvisation of workouts is all about.

- ➢ Maximum of 10 repetitions for any workouts (dumbbell/barbell) is enough for a single set. Once you find doing 10 repetitions more easy, it means it's time to increase weight.

Valuable Insights

➢ Endurance training/aerobics compliments weight training and vice versa.

➢ Carbohydrates and fats are as vital as proteins for gaining muscles.

➢ The workouts/diet ratio for building muscles is 50:50

➢ Non-vegetarian source of quality proteins will be more advantageous than vegetarian source of proteins. As they contain more amino acids than vegetarian source.

➢ Swimming and Yoga are useful to keep your muscles flexible and rejuvenated. And also for destressing the mind and stimulating appetite.

Motivational Quotes

A) Courage is the price life exacts for granting peace.

B) When your desires are strong enough, you will appear to possess super human powers to achieve.

C) The mind works through pictures. Pictures affect your self-image and your self-image affects the way you feel, act and achieve.

D) Success on the outside means nothing unless you also have success within. There is a huge difference between well-being and being well-off.

E) There is a bright side to the darkest circumstance, if you have the courage to look for it.

F) The secret of happiness is simple, find out what you truly love to do and then direct all your energy towards it.

G) Never do anything because you have to do it. The only reason to do something is because you want to and because you know it is the right thing for you to do.

H) Always remember that what lies behind you and what lies in front of you is nothing when compared to what lies within you.

I) The science of physicality is based on the principle that says as you care for the body so you care for the mind. As you prepare your body so you prepare your mind. As you train your body, so you train your mind.

J) Read regularly. Reading for thirty minutes a day will do wonders for you. All the mistakes you will ever make in your life have already been made by those that have walked before you. Every answer to every problem you have ever faced is in print. Read the right books.

K) Act in a way that is congruent with your true character. Be guided by your heart. Do the right things. Act with integrity. The rest will take care of itself.

L) Many lack a key ingredient to a meaningful enlightened life, the freedom to see the forest beyond trees, the freedom to choose what is right over what seems pressing.

M) Confidence doesn't come out of nowhere, it's a result of something...hours and days and weeks and years of constant work and dedication.

N) If we all worked on the assumption that what is accepted as true is really true, there would be little hope for advance.

O) Without a struggle, there can be no progress.

P) Physical fitness is not only the most important keys to a healthy body, it is the basis for dynamic and creative intellectual activity.

Q) Life is either a daring adventure or nothing at all.

R) Whatever you can do, or dream you can, begin it. Boldness has genius, power and magic in it.

S) There isn't a person anywhere who isn't capable of doing more than he thinks he can.

T) Life doesn't require that we be the best – only that we try our best.

U) I will do strongly before the sun and moon whatever inly rejoices me and the heart appoints.

Motivational Quotes

V) That which doesn't kill you, will make you stronger.

W) You cannot push a man beyond the definitions he holds in his mind.

X) To live, is to live fearlessly.

Y) Death is not the greatest loss in life. Loss in when life dies inside you while you are alive.

Z) Defeat is not when you fall down, It is when you refuse to get up.